Toxic Family 365
5 Minutes a Day to Toxic Family Healing
Steven Todd Bryant

Disclaimer

This book is not intended as a substitute for the medical advice of physicians. The reader must consult a physician in matters relating to his/her/their health and particularly with respect to any symptoms that may require diagnosis or medical attention. Although the author has made every effort to ensure the information in this book was correct at press time, the author does not assume and hereby disclaims any liability to any party for any loss, damage, or disruption caused by errors or omissions for any reason. The author cannot be held legally responsible for any damages suffered because of this publication or the content of 3rd party web pages or resources. In some cases, stories have been fictionalized, and names and identifying details have been omitted or changed to protect the privacy of individuals.

Table of Contents

About the Author

Steven Todd Bryant is a best-selling author, crisis counselor, toxic family survivor, and founder of ToxicFamily.org. He was on staff at the University of Southern California for 19 years and holds an MA in theological studies. He lives in Southern California.

Follow Steven Todd Bryant:
www.facebook.com/steventoddbryant
amazon.com/author/steventoddbryant
www.steventoddbryant.com/

Other Books by Steven Todd Bryant on Amazon:
The Toxic Family Solution
Unclutter Your Life to Find Meaning & Purpose
The Wisdom of Swedish Death Cleaning
Jesus & the LGBTQ Christian

Dedication

For Marcus, who inspired and motivated me during the writing of this book.

Do you feel trapped by the toxic dynamics of your family? Are you struggling with the emotional scars left by abusive or neglectful relationships? Maybe you've experienced symptoms like anxiety, depression, or low self-esteem, and you can't seem to break free from the grip of your past. The pain and confusion caused by toxic family members can be overwhelming and leave you feeling hopeless and lost.

Welcome to "Toxic Family 365: 5 Minutes a Day to Toxic Family Healing." This book is your holistic guide to breaking free from the chains of toxic family dynamics. It provides daily affirmations, reflections, and practical exercises to help you heal from past wounds, build resilience, and reclaim your life. It offers a step-by-step approach to understanding, coping with, and overcoming the harmful effects of toxic family relationships.

I know the depths of this struggle firsthand. For eighteen years, I lived in a domestically violent home where verbal, emotional, psychological, and spiritual abuse occurred daily. My father's parenting was a reign of terror, and although my mother showed love, she excused and enabled his destructive behavior. Despite moving away and achieving professional success, I carried the emotional baggage of my past. Through extensive therapy, personal development, and years of trial and error, I found a path to healing. I founded ToxicFamily.org to share my journey and help others find freedom from their toxic family dynamics.

This book will help you understand toxic family behaviors, set boundaries, practice self-care, and rebuild your self-esteem. Each month focuses on different themes, such as coping strategies, forgiveness, and living authentically. By following this year-long program, you will gain the tools to manage your emotions, develop healthier relationships, and create a life that reflects your true self.

The principles and strategies in this book are not just theoretical —they are practical solutions that have transformed my life and the lives of many others. Through my work as a crisis counselor and founder of ToxicFamily.org, I've seen firsthand how these methods can lead to profound healing and growth.

If you commit to reading this book and applying its principles, your life will change dramatically. You will break free from the emotional chains of your toxic family, rediscover your self-worth, and begin living the authentic, fulfilling life you deserve. Imagine waking up each day feeling empowered, confident, and free from the past. This book promises to be your roadmap to a brighter future.

Are you ready to transform your life and break free from the grip of your toxic family? Let's begin your 365-day journey to healing and empowerment. Each page holds the key to understanding your past, overcoming your pain, and building a future filled with joy and authenticity. Don't let another day go by feeling trapped and overwhelmed by your past. The longer you wait, the deeper these wounds can become. Time alone does not heal toxic family wounds—action does. Start your healing journey today and take the first step toward a healthier, happier life.

This book is designed to guide you on a year-long journey of healing and growth. Each month centers on a specific theme related to overcoming toxic family dynamics and building a healthier life. Within each month, weekly topics explore powerful subtopics, offering practical advice, insights, and exercises.

The affirmations, reflections, and exercises contained in this book are powerful tools for personal growth and healing. I know this firsthand—they changed my life! As a crisis counselor, I've also seen many others use these same techniques to create happier, brighter futures. These tools help reframe negative thoughts, reinforce positive beliefs, and encourage self-awareness. Each day's message includes an affirmation to inspire you, a reflection to help you explore your thoughts and feelings, and practical exercises designed to guide you toward greater self-compassion, resilience, and empowerment.

Monthly Themes Overview

January: Understanding Toxic Families – Learn about the characteristics and dynamics of toxic families and how they affect your well-being.

February: Coping with Your Toxic Family – Discover strategies for managing interactions with toxic family members while protecting your mental health.

March: When to Cut Ties and Walk Away – Explore the difficult decision of cutting ties with toxic family members and the steps involved.

April: Boundaries and Healthy Relationships – Understand the importance of setting boundaries and building healthy relationships.

May: Self-Care and Recovery – Focus on self-care practices and recovery techniques to heal from past trauma.

June: Getting Help When Needed – Learn about seeking professional support and utilizing resources to aid your healing journey.

July: Stop Toxic Thinking – Identify and challenge toxic thought patterns that hinder your growth.

August: Rebuilding Self-Esteem – Work on rebuilding your self-esteem and fostering self-love.

September: Creating a Support System – Understand the importance of a support system and how to build and maintain one.

October: Forgiveness and Letting Go – Explore the power of forgiveness and the process of letting go of past hurts.

November: Living Your Authentic Life – Embrace your true self and live authentically.

December: Continuing the Healing Journey – Reflect on your progress and set intentions for continued growth and healing.

I recommend you read through the entire book one time to familiarize yourself with the topics you will be addressing over the next year. After completing this initial read-through, you can begin your daily practice by starting with the current calendar day.

Embarking on a journey of healing from toxic family dynamics can be challenging, but it is also incredibly rewarding. Remember that progress may be slow at times, and setbacks are a natural part of the process. Be patient with yourself and celebrate every step forward, no matter how small. This book is here to support you, offering daily encouragement and practical guidance to help you stay motivated and focused on your goals.

As you begin this journey, know that you are not alone. Many others have faced similar challenges and found strength and resilience along the way. Use this book as a companion and guide, drawing on the wisdom and experiences shared within its pages. Together, we will work toward healing, growth, and the creation of a healthier, more fulfilling life. Welcome to "Toxic Family 365: 5 Minutes a Day to Toxic Family Healing"—your path to emotional freedom and empowerment starts now.

Best wishes and peace on your healing journey,

Steven Todd Bryant
Summer, 2024

January: Understanding Toxic Families

The first step in overcoming the impact of a toxic family is understanding the dynamics at play. Toxic families often involve patterns of behavior that are detrimental to individual well-being, such as manipulation, control, and emotional abuse. This month, we will look into what makes a family toxic, examining the common behaviors and traits found in such families and the profound effects these dynamics can have on one's mental, emotional, and even physical health.

Toxic family dynamics can be insidious, often masquerading as normalcy due to their persistent nature. They may include constant criticism, unrealistic expectations, neglect, emotional manipulation, and even outright abuse. Recognizing these behaviors is crucial because they can deeply affect your self-esteem, relationships, and overall mental health. By identifying these toxic patterns, you gain the power to confront and change them.

Throughout this month, we will explore the various types of toxic family behaviors. Manipulation can take many forms, from guilt-tripping and gaslighting to more subtle forms of emotional coercion. Control often manifests as micromanaging, excessive demands, and a lack of respect for personal boundaries. Emotional abuse, perhaps the most damaging, can include verbal assaults, emotional neglect, and constant belittlement.

We will also examine the roles that individuals within toxic families often play. Understanding these roles can provide insight into the dysfunctional dynamics and help you see the bigger picture of how each person's behavior contributes to the overall toxicity. For instance, the roles of the enabler, the scapegoat, the golden child, and the lost child each have distinct characteristics and impacts on family dynamics.

The effects of growing up in or being part of a toxic family can be long-lasting and far-reaching. They can lead to issues such as chronic anxiety, depression, low self-esteem, trust issues, and difficulties in forming healthy relationships. Physical health can also be impacted, with stress-related illnesses being a common consequence. Understanding these effects is a vital step in acknowledging your pain and starting your healing journey.

By gaining a clearer understanding of these issues, you will be better equipped to recognize toxic patterns and begin the journey toward healing. Knowledge is indeed power. The more you understand about the nature of toxic families, the better you can navigate your own experiences and set the foundation for a healthier future. This month, commit to gaining the insights needed to see your family dynamics with fresh, informed eyes. This knowledge will empower you to take meaningful steps toward recovery and reclaiming your life.

Week 1: Identifying a Toxic Family

Introduction of Week's Theme

Recognizing the signs of a toxic family is a critical first step toward breaking free from its harmful influence and reclaiming your well-being. Toxic family dynamics can be deeply ingrained and often disguised as everyday interactions, making them challenging to identify without a clear understanding of their characteristics. This week, we will focus on identifying the specific traits and behaviors that typify toxic family environments, providing you with the tools to see your situation with greater clarity and validation.

Understanding the hallmarks of toxic family dynamics is essential because these patterns can subtly erode your self-esteem, sense of security, and overall mental health. Common signs of a toxic family include constant criticism, where family members may belittle or undermine you regularly, making you feel inadequate or unworthy. This pervasive negativity can leave lasting emotional scars and foster a deep sense of self-doubt.

Another significant indicator is the lack of boundaries. In toxic families, personal boundaries are often disregarded or violated, leading to feelings of intrusion and loss of autonomy. This can manifest in various ways, such as disrespecting privacy, imposing unrealistic demands, or controlling aspects of your life that should be your own to decide. Recognizing the importance of boundaries and identifying when they are being crossed is crucial for your emotional well-being.

Emotional manipulation is another common trait in toxic families. This can include guilt-tripping, where you are made to feel responsible for others' happiness or problems, and emotional blackmail, where affection or approval is conditional based on your compliance with their expectations. Gaslighting, a particularly insidious form of manipulation, involves making you question your reality and perceptions, often leading to confusion, self-doubt, and a diminished sense of self-worth.

Throughout this week, we will explore these behaviors in detail, helping you to identify them in your own family dynamics. By understanding these signs, you can begin to validate your feelings and experiences, acknowledging that the pain and confusion you may feel are not your fault. This awareness is a powerful tool for breaking free from the toxic influence and starting your journey toward healing.

Embrace this week as an opportunity to gain a deeper understanding of your family dynamics and validate your experiences. As you progress through the week, remember that recognizing these signs is not about assigning blame but about gaining clarity and understanding. It's about empowering yourself with the knowledge to see your situation more objectively and take proactive steps toward a healthier, more fulfilling life. Your feelings and experiences are valid, and by identifying the toxic patterns in your family, you are taking the first vital step in reclaiming your life and well-being.

January 1

- **Affirmation:** "I am worthy of a loving and supportive family environment."
- **Reflection:** "A healthy family supports and nurtures its members. If you feel constantly drained or hurt by your family interactions, it may be a sign of toxicity."
- **Practical Exercise:** Write down three behaviors from your family that make you feel uncomfortable or hurt. Reflect on how these behaviors impact your well-being.

January 2

- **Affirmation:** "I trust my instincts and recognize when something feels wrong."
- **Reflection:** "Your gut feelings are valuable indicators of unhealthy dynamics. Pay attention to them."
- **Practical Exercise:** Think of a recent family interaction where you felt uneasy. Write about what happened and how it made you feel.

January 3

- **Affirmation:** "I deserve to have my feelings and experiences validated."
- **Reflection:** "Toxic families often dismiss or invalidate your emotions. Recognize that your feelings are valid and important."
- **Practical Exercise:** Share your feelings about a family issue with a trusted friend or therapist and note their

response. Compare it to your family's typical reaction.

January 4

- **Affirmation:** "I can identify manipulative behaviors and protect myself from them."
- **Reflection:** "Manipulation often involves guilt-tripping, gaslighting, and emotional blackmail. Being aware of these tactics is the first step to countering them."
- **Practical Exercise:** List common manipulative phrases you hear from your family. Next to each, write a counter-statement that reaffirms your autonomy and self-worth.

January 5

- **Affirmation:** "I acknowledge the impact of toxic behavior on my mental health."
- **Reflection:** "Recognizing the harm done by toxic family dynamics is essential for healing. It's not your fault."
- **Practical Exercise:** Journal about a time when a family member's behavior negatively impacted your mental health. Reflect on how acknowledging this impact makes you feel.

January 6

- **Affirmation:** "I recognize and honor the wounds I carry from my past."
- **Reflection:** "Acknowledging your wounds is not a sign of weakness but a step toward healing."
- **Practical Exercise:** Identify and write about a specific wound you carry from your family. How has it affected you over the years?

January 7

- **Affirmation:** "My pain is real, and I am allowed to grieve my past."
- **Reflection:** "Grieving the loss of a nurturing family is a natural and necessary part of healing."
- **Practical Exercise:** Write a letter to your younger self, acknowledging their pain and offering compassion

and support.

Week 2: Wounds Caused by Toxic Families

Introduction of Week's Theme

The emotional and psychological wounds caused by toxic families can be profound, deep-rooted, and long-lasting. These wounds shape our perceptions, influence our behaviors, and affect our overall mental and emotional health. This week, we will explore the various types of wounds that often result from growing up in a toxic family, including abandonment, betrayal, and chronic stress. Understanding these wounds is a crucial step toward healing and rebuilding your sense of self-worth.

Abandonment wounds arise when a family member, often a parent, is physically or emotionally absent. This absence can lead to feelings of neglect, loneliness, and a pervasive fear of being left behind. The impact of abandonment can manifest in adult relationships, where you might fear intimacy or constantly seek validation from others to fill the void left by the absent family member.

Betrayal wounds occur when trust is broken by those who are supposed to protect and nurture you. This could involve instances of deceit, broken promises, or acts of harm. Betrayal can leave you feeling vulnerable and mistrustful, making it challenging to form healthy, trusting relationships in the future. Understanding the roots of betrayal can help you start the process of rebuilding trust and learning to protect yourself from further harm.

Chronic stress is another significant wound inflicted by toxic family dynamics. Constant exposure to conflict, unpredictability, and emotional turmoil can lead to a state of heightened anxiety and hyper-vigilance. This state of constant alertness can exhaust your mental and physical resources, leading to issues such as insomnia, chronic fatigue, and stress-related illnesses. Recognizing the impact of chronic stress is vital to addressing its effects and finding ways to bring calm and balance back into your life.

In addition to these primary wounds, toxic family environments can also cause feelings of guilt, shame, and unworthiness. You might internalize the negative messages from your family, leading to a persistent inner critic that undermines your self-esteem and confidence. These feelings can be pervasive, affecting every aspect of your life, from personal relationships to professional endeavors.

Healing these wounds is not an overnight process, but it is a journey worth undertaking. Additionally, you may decide to seek the help of a trained therapist to guide you through overcoming the effects of any toxic family trauma you may be experiencing.

As you explore the nature and impact of your wounds, remember that you are taking the first steps toward reclaiming your power and rebuilding your sense of self-worth. You deserve to live a life free from the shadows of your past, and understanding your wounds is the key to unlocking that future.

This week, commit to facing your wounds with self-compassion and courage. Allow yourself to fully experience the emotions that arise, trusting that this process will lead to greater healing and self-empowerment. Embrace this opportunity to work through the layers of pain and begin to uncover the resilient, worthy individual that lies just beneath the surface. You are amazing. You are worthy of love and happiness.

January 8
- **Affirmation:** "I can heal from the emotional scars left by my toxic family."
- **Reflection:** "Healing is possible, and it begins with acknowledging the hurt and taking steps to recover."
- **Practical Exercise:** Research and list three healing

practices (e.g., therapy, support groups, mindfulness) that resonate with you. Plan how you can incorporate one into your life.

January 9

- **Affirmation:** "I will not let my past define my future."
- **Reflection:** "While your past has shaped you, it does not have to dictate your future. You have the power to create a new path."
- **Practical Exercise:** Visualize a future where you have healed from your past wounds. Write down what this future looks like and how it feels.

January 10

- **Affirmation:** "I am stronger than the pain I have endured."
- **Reflection:** "Your resilience is a testament to your strength. Embrace it as you move forward."
- **Practical Exercise:** Reflect on a time when you demonstrated resilience in the face of adversity. Write about what you learned from that experience.

January 11

- **Affirmation:** "I am not alone in my journey; support is available."
- **Reflection:** "Seeking help is a sign of strength, not weakness. Recognize the importance of support."
- **Practical Exercise:** Identify one supportive resource you can reach out to, such as a therapist, support group, or trusted friend. Make a plan to connect with them.

January 12

- **Affirmation:** "I forgive myself for the mistakes I made while trying to survive."
- **Reflection:** "Self-forgiveness is a crucial part of healing. Allow yourself to be human."
- **Practical Exercise:** Write a letter of forgiveness to yourself, acknowledging the mistakes you've made and expressing compassion and understanding.

January 13
- **Affirmation:** "I deserve to heal and be happy."
- **Reflection:** "Your happiness and well-being are worth striving for. Believe in your right to heal."
- **Practical Exercise:** List three things that bring you joy and commit to incorporating them into your week.

January 14
- **Affirmation:** "I release the negative emotions tied to my past."
- **Reflection:** "Holding onto negative emotions can hinder your healing. Learn to let go."
- **Practical Exercise:** Engage in a physical activity, like yoga or a walk in nature, to help release pent-up emotions. Reflect on how it feels to let go.

Week 3: Gaslighting and Emotional Manipulation

Introduction of Week's Theme

Gaslighting and emotional manipulation are insidious tactics often employed in toxic families to undermine your perception of reality and exert control over your behavior. These manipulative strategies can leave you doubting your own thoughts, feelings, and memories, causing significant psychological and emotional distress. This week, we will look into the nature of gaslighting and emotional manipulation, providing you with the tools and insights necessary to recognize, counter, and protect yourself from these harmful behaviors.

Gaslighting is a form of abuse toxic family members use to control and manipulate their loved ones. Gaslighting occurs when the parent or family member tries to cause the victim to question their sanity, perception of reality, or memories of what happened. The term originated from a 1944 film called *Gaslight*, where a husband tried to convince his wife she imagined things to drive her insane and control her behavior. Gaslighters will create a false narrative to shift the blame for what happened from themselves onto someone or something else. In some cases, gaslighters attempt to convince their victims that what they remember never happened or the abuse they experienced was not as severe as they recall.

The following are examples of gaslighting statements:
- "Can't you take a joke?"
- "Don't be so dramatic."
- "I'm sorry you think that's what happened."
- "I never did/said that."
- "It didn't happen like that."
- "It didn't really hurt."
- "That's not what happened."
- "You're crazy."
- "You're just imagining things."
- "You're overreacting."
- "You're making a big deal over nothing."
- "You're remembering it wrong."
- "You're too sensitive."
- "You're totally misinterpreting what is happening."

Gaslighting involves deliberately making someone question their own reality, often by denying the truth, twisting facts, or dismissing the victim's experiences and feelings. This tactic can be incredibly disorienting and damaging, leading to a loss of confidence and self-trust. Emotional manipulation, on the other hand, encompasses a range of behaviors aimed at controlling or influencing your emotions and actions to serve the manipulator's agenda. These behaviors can include guilt-tripping, emotional blackmail, silent treatment, and feigned victimhood.

Reclaiming your sense of reality is vital to countering gaslighting and emotional manipulation. This involves reaffirming your perceptions, trusting your instincts, and seeking validation from trusted sources outside of the toxic family environment. By strengthening your emotional resilience and fortifying your sense of self, you can effectively shield yourself from the harmful effects of gaslighting and emotional manipulation.

As you navigate through this week's lessons, remember that recognizing and addressing these toxic behaviors is a significant step toward healing and empowerment. You have the right to your own reality, your own feelings, and your own life. By reclaiming your sense of reality and protecting yourself from manipulation, you are taking powerful strides toward a healthier, more authentic existence.

When it comes to gaslighting and emotional manipulation, always trust your intuition and feelings. Let your heart be your guide to what is true. Gaslighters thrive on making you doubt your reality and sense of self, but your inner voice knows the truth. Pay attention to the subtle signals your body and emotions send you when something feels off.

Trusting your instincts can help you navigate through the confusion and deceit, allowing you to see situations and people for who they truly are. Remember, your feelings are valid, and honoring them is a crucial step toward maintaining your mental and emotional well-being.

If your heart tells you that your family is unhealthy, believe it. Maya Angelou wrote, "When someone shows you who they are, believe them the first time."

January 15
- **Affirmation:** "I trust my perception of reality."
- **Reflection:** "Gaslighting is designed to make you doubt your perceptions. Reaffirming your reality is crucial."
- **Practical Exercise:** Write about a situation where you felt gaslighted. Describe what actually happened and how it made you feel.

January 16

- **Affirmation:** "I can recognize manipulative behaviors and respond assertively."
- **Reflection:** "Being able to identify manipulation is the first step to resisting it."
- **Practical Exercise:** Role-play with a friend or therapist how to respond to manipulative statements assertively.

January 17

- **Affirmation:** "My feelings and experiences are valid."
- **Reflection:** "Emotional manipulators often invalidate your feelings. Stand firm in your truth."
- **Practical Exercise:** List instances when your feelings were invalidated. Write affirmations that validate your experiences.

January 18

- **Affirmation:** "I will set boundaries to protect myself from emotional manipulation."
- **Reflection:** "Boundaries are essential for safeguarding your emotional well-being." For example, one might tell someone who is gaslighting them, " My interpretation of what happened is valid and deserves respect."
- **Practical Exercise:** Identify a boundary you need to set with a family member and plan how to communicate it clearly.

January 19

- **Affirmation:** "I have the power to reject manipulation and stand firm in my truth."
- **Reflection:** "Rejecting manipulation involves recognizing it and affirming your reality."
- **Practical Exercise:** Practice affirming your truth in front of a mirror. Rehearse how you will respond to a common manipulative tactic you face.

January 20

- **Affirmation:** "I deserve to be treated with respect and

honesty."
   - **Reflection:** "Respect and honesty are fundamental to healthy relationships. Demand them."
   - **Practical Exercise:** Reflect on your relationships and identify which ones respect your boundaries and honesty. Consider how you can strengthen these relationships and distance yourself from those that do not.

January 21
   - **Affirmation:** "I am resilient and capable of protecting myself."
   - **Reflection:** "Your resilience is a powerful tool in combating manipulation. Trust in your strength."
   - **Practical Exercise:** Write about a time when you successfully stood up for yourself. Reflect on the strategies you used and how they made you feel.

Week 4: Roles That Hinder Self-Expression

Introduction of Week's Theme

In toxic families, individuals are often unconsciously assigned specific roles that limit their ability to express their true selves and thrive. These roles can be deeply ingrained, shaping behaviors, thoughts, and interactions in ways that suppress individuality and personal growth. This week, we will focus on identifying these roles, understanding how they hinder self-expression, and learning how to break free from their constraints.

Toxic family roles often serve to maintain a dysfunctional equilibrium, preventing the family system from facing and addressing underlying issues. Typical roles include the enabler, who supports the toxic behavior of others; the scapegoat, who is blamed for the family's problems; the golden child, who is idealized and burdened with unrealistic expectations; and the lost child, who is ignored and overlooked. Each of these roles comes with its own set of challenges and limitations.

Understanding these roles is crucial because they dictate how family members interact with each other and the outside world. The enabler often sacrifices their own needs to keep the peace, suppressing their emotions and desires. The scapegoat internalizes blame and criticism, leading to low self-esteem and self-doubt. The golden child may feel immense pressure to live up to impossible standards, stifling their true interests and passions and causing them to struggle with perfectionism. The lost child, in their effort to avoid conflict, may become disconnected from their own feelings and aspirations.

Throughout this week, we will explore the characteristics and behaviors associated with each role. By recognizing these patterns in your own life, you can begin to understand how they have shaped your self-perception and interactions. We will explore how these roles are assigned, often unconsciously, and how they perpetuate a cycle of dysfunction and suppression.

Breaking free from these roles involves a multifaceted approach. It starts with awareness—acknowledging the role you have been assigned and its impact on your life. From there, we will work on strategies to reclaim your individuality and voice. This includes setting boundaries, practicing self-compassion, and redefining your identity outside of the family's expectations.

January 22
- **Affirmation:** "I am more than the role my family assigned to me."
- **Reflection:** "Toxic families often box individuals into restrictive roles. Recognize that you are multifaceted."
- **Practical Exercise:** Write about the role you were assigned in your family and how it has limited your self-expression.

January 23
- **Affirmation:** "I have the right to express my true self."
- **Reflection:** "Self-expression is a fundamental human

right. Embrace it."
- **Practical Exercise:** Engage in an activity that allows you to express yourself freely (e.g., art, writing, music). Reflect on how it feels.

January 24
- **Affirmation:** "I reject the labels that limit me."
- **Reflection:** "Labels from toxic families can be confining. Reject them and embrace your true identity."
- **Practical Exercise:** List the labels your family has given you. Write counter-statements that affirm your true qualities and strengths.

January 25
- **Affirmation:** "I can redefine my identity on my terms."
- **Reflection:** "You have the power to define who you are, independent of your family's expectations."
- **Practical Exercise:** Write a personal mission statement that reflects your true values and aspirations. A personal mission statement is a concise declaration of your core values, guiding principles, and aspirations, serving as a blueprint for living an authentic and purposeful life.

January 26
- **Affirmation:** "I will pursue my passions and interests."
- **Reflection:** "Your passions and interests are a vital part of your identity. Pursue them with confidence."
- **Practical Exercise:** Identify a passion or interest that you have neglected due to family pressures. Make a plan to incorporate it into your life.

January 27
- **Affirmation:** "I deserve to be seen and heard for who I truly am."
- **Reflection:** "Being seen and heard is essential for a healthy sense of self."
- **Practical Exercise:** Share something meaningful about yourself with a trusted friend or group. Notice how it feels to be acknowledged.

January 28
- **Affirmation:** "I have the courage to break free from toxic roles."
- **Reflection:** "Breaking free from toxic roles requires courage and determination. You can do it."
- **Practical Exercise:** Identify one step you can take today to challenge the role you've been assigned. Take that step and reflect on the experience.

January 29
- **Affirmation:** "I am worthy of love and respect just as I am."
- **Reflection:** "Your worth is intrinsic and not defined by the roles others assign to you."
- **Practical Exercise:** Write a letter to yourself affirming your worth and the qualities you love about yourself.

January 30
- **Affirmation:** "I will nurture my authentic self."
- **Reflection:** "Nurturing your true self is vital for personal growth and fulfillment."
- **Practical Exercise:** Spend time each day this week doing something that genuinely makes you happy and reflects your true self.

January 31
- **Affirmation:** "I am proud of my progress and my journey towards self-expression."
- **Reflection:** "Acknowledge and celebrate your journey and the progress you've made."
- **Practical Exercise:** Reflect on the changes you have made this month and celebrate your progress in a meaningful way.

January Conclusion

As we conclude this month's focus on understanding toxic families, take a moment to reflect on the profound knowledge and insights you have gained. Recognizing the signs of toxic behavior, understanding the wounds they cause, and learning to identify and counter manipulation are foundational steps in your healing journey. These lessons are not merely academic; they are tools of empowerment that will guide you toward a healthier, more fulfilling life.

Throughout January, you have embarked on a transformative journey of self-discovery and awareness. By exploring the dynamics of toxic families, you have begun to dismantle the harmful patterns that have impacted your life. You have learned to trust your instincts, validate your feelings, and recognize your worth. This understanding is a powerful catalyst for change, enabling you to break free from the harmful influences of your past.

Embracing your true self and breaking free from restrictive roles is a courageous act of self-love and self-affirmation. You are reclaiming your identity, not as defined by your family's expectations, but as defined by your values, passions, and dreams. This reclamation is a significant step toward living a life that is authentically yours.

The journey of healing is ongoing and requires patience, compassion, and an unwavering commitment to yourself. Healing is not linear; it involves progress and setbacks, but each step, no matter how small, is a victory worth celebrating. Acknowledge the strength and resilience you have demonstrated. Each boundary set, each moment of self-care, and each act of self-compassion is a testament to your courage and determination.

Celebrate the progress you have made so far. Reflect on the victories, big and small, that you have achieved. You are resilient, strong, and worthy of every step you take toward healing and self-discovery. Each milestone, no matter how small, is a testament to your courage and determination. Embrace your journey with pride, knowing that you have the power to create a life filled with peace, joy, and fulfillment. Keep moving forward. You have greatness within you!

February: Coping with Your Toxic Family

Coping with a toxic family can be an ongoing challenge, especially when complete separation is not an option. The emotional turmoil, stress, and negativity that toxic family dynamics create can significantly impact your mental health and overall well-being. This month, we will focus on practical and effective strategies to manage your interactions with toxic family members while safeguarding your mental and emotional health.

By learning how to navigate these difficult relationships, you can minimize their impact on your life and create a more supportive environment. We will explore various coping mechanisms that can help you maintain your sanity and emotional balance, even in the face of persistent negativity. These strategies will empower you to handle difficult situations with confidence and resilience.

We will explore practical ways to cope with the stress and negativity that often accompany toxic family dynamics, emphasizing the importance of self-care and setting boundaries. Self-care is not a luxury; it is a necessity for maintaining your mental health. Establishing clear and firm boundaries is crucial to protect yourself from the emotional fallout that often comes with toxic relationships.

Remember, you have the power to protect your well-being and

take control of your interactions. Coping with a toxic family is not about changing them; it's about changing how you respond to them. By developing these healthier ways of coping, you can reclaim your power and create a sense of stability and peace in your life.

Week 1: Strategies for Spending Time with Unhealthy Families

Introduction of Week's Theme

Spending time with unhealthy families can be challenging and emotionally draining. It's crucial to have effective strategies in place to protect your emotional and mental well-being. By developing a toolkit of coping mechanisms, you can reduce stress, set clear boundaries, and maintain your sense of self when dealing with toxic family members.

We will explore practical techniques for managing difficult conversations, establishing and enforcing personal boundaries, and finding healthy ways to detach emotionally when necessary. Additionally, we'll consider the importance of self-care practices to replenish your energy and maintain your mental health after spending time with your family. Understanding and implementing these strategies can significantly improve your ability to handle toxic dynamics, allowing you to engage with family on your terms while prioritizing your well-being.

February 1

- **Affirmation:** "I will prioritize my well-being in all interactions with my family."
- **Reflection:** "Your well-being is paramount. Make decisions that support your mental and emotional health."
- **Practical Exercise:** Plan an upcoming family interaction. Set clear boundaries for what you are willing to tolerate and decide on exit strategies if the situation becomes overwhelming.

February 2

- **Affirmation:** "I can control my reactions, even if I cannot control others' actions."
- **Reflection:** "You have the power to choose how you respond to toxic behavior."
- **Practical Exercise:** Reflect on a recent family conflict. Identify how you reacted and how you could respond more constructively in the future.

February 3

- **Affirmation:** "I will stay grounded and centered during family interactions."
- **Reflection:** "Staying grounded helps you maintain your composure and protect your emotional state."
- **Practical Exercise:** Practice deep breathing or grounding exercises before and during family interactions. Notice the difference it makes in how you handle stress.

February 4

- **Affirmation:** "I will not let my family's negativity define my self-worth."
- **Reflection:** "Others' opinions or behaviors do not determine your value."
- **Practical Exercise:** Write a list of positive affirmations about yourself. Repeat them before and after family interactions to reinforce your self-worth.

February 5

- **Affirmation:** "I can create a positive environment for myself, even in challenging situations."
- **Reflection:** "You have the power to influence your environment and bring positivity into your life."
- **Practical Exercise:** Identify ways to bring positivity into your interactions. This could be through setting a positive tone, redirecting negative conversations, or taking breaks when needed.

February 6

- **Affirmation:** "I will assertively communicate my

boundaries."
- **Reflection:** "Clear and assertive communication of boundaries helps protect your well-being."
- **Practical Exercise:** Write down a boundary you need to communicate to a family member. Practice how you will assertively convey this boundary in a calm and clear manner.

February 7
- **Affirmation:** "I am deserving of respect and consideration."
- **Reflection:** "Respect and consideration are fundamental to healthy interactions. Demand them."
- **Practical Exercise:** Reflect on a recent interaction where you felt disrespected. Plan how you will address this issue and assert your need for respectful treatment in future interactions.

Week 2: Healthy Coping Behaviors

Introduction of Week's Theme

Developing healthy coping behaviors is essential for managing the stress and emotional turmoil that comes from dealing with a toxic family. Unhealthy coping mechanisms, such as substance abuse, emotional eating, or self-isolation, can exacerbate your stress and prolong your suffering. This week, we will explore various strategies and practices that can help you cope in healthier ways, ensuring that you protect your well-being and maintain a balanced life.

Here are some examples of healthy coping mechanisms:

- **Exercise**: Engaging in physical activity to reduce stress and improve mental health.
- **Mindfulness**: Practicing mindfulness techniques such as meditation or deep breathing to stay present and manage anxiety.
- **Creative Expression**: Expressing emotions through

art, music, writing, or other creative outlets.

- **Social Support**: Seeking connection and support from friends, family, or support groups to share experiences and gain perspective.
- **Healthy Eating**: Maintaining a balanced diet to support overall well-being and manage stress effectively.

Healthy coping behaviors are vital for not only surviving but thriving despite the challenges posed by toxic family dynamics. These behaviors empower you to handle difficult emotions constructively, reduce stress, and build resilience. We will explore techniques such as mindfulness, physical activity, creative expression, and social connection, all of which can play a significant role in enhancing your emotional and mental health.

By adopting these healthy coping strategies, you will learn to navigate the complexities of your family relationships without compromising your own well-being. We will also examine the importance of self-compassion and self-care and how integrating these practices into your daily routine can provide a solid foundation for emotional stability.

Mindfulness is a healthy coping mechanism because it encourages living in the present moment, allowing you to observe your thoughts and emotions as if from afar and without judgment. By practicing mindfulness, you can create a safe space and gain distance from troubling thoughts, emotions, and behavior of others. With mindfulness, you can create a sense of calm and clarity, which helps in reducing stress and anxiety.

Mindfulness can help you cultivate a deeper connection with yourself, enabling you to recognize and address negative thought patterns and emotional triggers more effectively. Mindfulness exercises, such as meditation and mindful breathing, can enhance your tolerance for stress, improve your focus, and cultivate a balanced and peaceful mind, making them essential tools for navigating life's challenges gracefully and peacefully.

February 8
- **Affirmation:** "I will practice self-care to nurture my mind, body, and spirit."
- **Reflection:** "Self-care is crucial for maintaining your overall well-being."
- **Practical Exercise:** Create a self-care plan that includes activities that nurture your mind, body, and spirit. Commit to incorporating these activities into your routine.

February 9
- **Affirmation:** "I will seek support from those who understand and uplift me."
- **Reflection:** "Supportive relationships are vital for your mental and emotional health."
- **Practical Exercise:** Reach out to a trusted friend or support group to share your experiences. Notice how their support and understanding impact your well-being.

February 10
- **Affirmation:** "I will engage in activities that bring me joy and relaxation."
- **Reflection:** "Finding joy and relaxation is essential for coping with stress."
- **Practical Exercise:** Identify activities that bring you joy and relaxation. Schedule time for at least one of these activities this week.

February 11
- **Affirmation:** "I will set realistic expectations for myself and my family."
- **Reflection:** "Setting realistic expectations helps you manage your responses and reduce disappointment."
- **Practical Exercise:** Reflect on your expectations of your family and yourself. Adjust them to be more

realistic and compassionate.

February 12
- **Affirmation:** "I will practice mindfulness to stay present and calm."
- **Reflection:** "Mindfulness helps you stay grounded and manage stress more effectively."
- **Practical Exercise:** Practice a mindfulness exercise, such as mindful breathing or meditation, to help you stay present and calm during stressful interactions.

February 13
- **Affirmation:** "I will prioritize healthy coping mechanisms over harmful ones."
- **Reflection:** "Choosing healthy coping mechanisms is a step toward long-term well-being."
- **Practical Exercise:** Identify one unhealthy coping mechanism you tend to use. Replace it with a healthier alternative and track your progress.

February 14
- **Affirmation:** "I deserve to take care of myself first."
- **Reflection:** "Self-care is not selfish; it is essential for your well-being."
- **Practical Exercise:** Dedicate time today to an activity that is solely for your enjoyment and relaxation. Reflect on how it feels to prioritize yourself.

Week 3: Unhealthy Coping Behaviors

Introduction of Week's Theme

Identifying and addressing unhealthy coping behaviors is crucial for your long-term well-being. These behaviors, while sometimes providing temporary relief, can ultimately exacerbate your stress and emotional pain, leading to a cycle of negativity and self-destruction. This week, we will explore the various unhealthy coping mechanisms that many people develop as a response to the stress and trauma of toxic family dynamics.

Here are some examples of unhealthy coping mechanisms:

- **Substance Abuse:** Using drugs or alcohol to escape or numb emotional pain.
- **Emotional Eating:** Turning to food for comfort, leading to overeating or unhealthy eating patterns.
- **Self-Isolation:** Withdrawing from social interactions and support systems.
- **Self-Harm:** Engaging in behaviors that inflict physical harm to oneself as a way to cope with emotional distress.
- **Procrastination:** Avoiding tasks or responsibilities, leading to increased stress and feelings of overwhelm.

Throughout this week, you are encouraged to identify the unhealthy coping mechanisms you may currently rely on and replace them with more positive alternatives. By making these changes, you can begin to break free from the negative patterns that have been holding you back and move toward a healthier, more fulfilling life.

Recognizing these behaviors is the first step toward change. It's essential to understand why you might turn to these coping mechanisms and how they affect your overall well-being. By becoming aware of the triggers and patterns that lead to these behaviors, you can start to break the cycle and pave the way for healthier habits.

February 15
- **Affirmation:** "I am aware of my coping mechanisms and strive to make healthier choices."
- **Reflection:** "Awareness is the first step toward change."
- **Practical Exercise:** Identify unhealthy coping behaviors you currently use. Write about why you turn to these behaviors and how they impact your life.

February 16

- **Affirmation:** "I can replace unhealthy habits with healthier ones."
- **Reflection:** "Changing your habits takes time and effort, but it's possible."
- **Practical Exercise:** Choose one unhealthy coping behavior to replace. Identify a healthier alternative and make a plan to implement it.

February 17

- **Affirmation:** "I am patient with myself as I work to change my habits."
- **Reflection:** "Changing habits is a process that requires patience and self-compassion."
- **Practical Exercise:** Reflect on your progress in changing unhealthy habits. Write about the challenges you face and how you can overcome them.

February 18

- **Affirmation:** "I will not use substances or food to numb my emotions."
- **Reflection:** "Using substances or food to cope can lead to more significant issues."
- **Practical Exercise:** Identify triggers that lead you to use substances or food for comfort. Develop alternative coping strategies for these triggers.

February 19

- **Affirmation:** "I deserve to treat myself with kindness and respect."
- **Reflection:** "Self-compassion is essential for overcoming unhealthy coping behaviors."
- **Practical Exercise:** Practice self-compassion by writing a letter to yourself, acknowledging your efforts to change and offering encouragement.

February 20

- **Affirmation:** "I can find healthier ways to cope with stress."
- **Reflection:** "Healthy coping mechanisms promote long-term well-being."
- **Practical Exercise:** Make a list of healthy coping

strategies that appeal to you. Choose one to try the next time you feel stressed.

February 21
- **Affirmation:** "I am in control of my actions and choices."
- **Reflection:** "You have the power to choose healthier ways to cope."
- **Practical Exercise:** Reflect on a recent situation where you used an unhealthy coping mechanism. Write about how you could handle a similar situation differently in the future.

Week 4: Coping with Negative Emotions

Introduction of Week's Theme

Negative emotions are a natural and inevitable response to difficult family dynamics. Feelings such as anger, sadness, fear, and frustration can be overwhelming when you are dealing with toxic family members. However, it is essential to understand that these emotions, while intense, do not have to dominate or control your life. This week, we will explore healthy and effective strategies for coping with and managing negative emotions.

By gaining a deeper understanding of your emotional responses, you can begin to process and release the hold they have on you. This week's theme focuses on developing practical techniques to handle negative emotions constructively, such as mindfulness practices, journaling, and breathing exercises.

We will also examine the importance of self-compassion and self-care in managing emotional health. Learning to recognize and validate your feelings is a critical step in healing, and finding ways to soothe and nurture yourself during emotional turmoil is equally vital. Additionally, we will discuss how to build and lean on a support system, including friends, support groups, and professionals who can offer guidance and comfort.

Remember, coping with negative emotions is not about suppressing or ignoring them but about acknowledging and processing them in a healthy way.

February 22

- **Affirmation:** "I acknowledge my negative emotions without judgment."
- **Reflection:** "It's okay to feel negative emotions. Acknowledging them is the first step to managing them."
- **Practical Exercise:** Write about a recent experience that elicited negative emotions. Acknowledge these feelings without judgment.

February 23

- **Affirmation:** "I will express my emotions in healthy and constructive ways."
- **Reflection:** "Expressing emotions healthily helps you process and release them."
- **Practical Exercise:** Choose a healthy way to express your emotions, such as journaling, talking to a friend, or engaging in physical activity. Practice this method this week.

February 24

- **Affirmation:** "I can transform my negative emotions into positive actions."
- **Reflection:** "Negative emotions can be powerful motivators for positive change."
- **Practical Exercise:** Identify a negative emotion you frequently experience. Find a way to channel this emotion into a positive action or project.

February 25

- **Affirmation:** "I will practice gratitude to balance my perspective."
- **Reflection:** "Gratitude helps shift your focus from negative to positive aspects of your life."
- **Practical Exercise:** Write a daily gratitude list for the next week. Note how this practice influences your

emotional state.

February 26
- **Affirmation:** "I will seek help when my emotions feel overwhelming."
- **Reflection:** "Seeking help is a sign of strength, not weakness."
- **Practical Exercise:** Identify resources for emotional support, such as a therapist, support group, or crisis hotline. Reach out to one of these resources if needed.

February 27
- **Affirmation:** "I am capable of managing my emotions in healthy ways."
- **Reflection:** "Believing in your ability to manage your emotions is crucial for success."
- **Practical Exercise:** Reflect on a time when you successfully managed a difficult emotion. Write about what you did and how it helped.

February 28
- **Affirmation:** "I will practice self-compassion during difficult emotional moments."
- **Reflection:** "Being kind to yourself when experiencing negative emotions fosters healing and growth."
- **Practical Exercise:** Write a self-compassionate response to a recent situation where you felt overwhelmed by negative emotions.

February Conclusion

As we conclude this month dedicated to coping with your toxic family, take a deep breath and truly acknowledge the significant progress you have made. This month we explored various aspects of coping with toxic family dynamics, starting with strategies for spending time with unhealthy family members. You have discovered ways to navigate interactions with toxic relatives while safeguarding your peace of mind. These strategies are not just practical tips but essential tools for maintaining your emotional stability and resilience in difficult environments.

Next, we explored healthy coping behaviors. You have learned to identify and implement positive coping mechanisms that nurture your mental and emotional health. Whether through mindfulness, exercise, or creative expression, you have found healthier ways to deal with stress and emotional turmoil. Each step you take in adopting these healthy habits is a victory on your path to recovery.

We also addressed unhealthy coping behaviors, helping you recognize and begin to replace them with more constructive alternatives. Acknowledging these behaviors and taking steps to change them is a courageous act of self-awareness and self-improvement. Celebrate each small victory, and be patient with yourself as you continue this transformation.

Finally, we focused on coping with negative emotions. By gaining a deeper understanding of your emotional responses, you have equipped yourself with the tools to manage and process these feelings constructively. Embracing techniques like mindfulness, journaling, and breathing exercises have empowered you to handle stress and maintain your composure even in the face of challenging family dynamics.

March: When to Cut Ties and Walk Away

Deciding when to cut ties with toxic family members is one of the most challenging and transformative decisions you may face. Toxic family dynamics can deeply impact your mental, emotional, and even physical well-being, often leaving you feeling trapped, powerless, and emotionally drained. The decision to sever ties is not taken lightly; it involves a profound recognition of the negative impact these relationships have on your life and a courageous commitment to prioritizing your health and happiness.

This month, we will examine the complexities of this decision and explore the specific circumstances that might necessitate walking away, such as chronic manipulation, emotional or physical abuse, and persistent boundary violations. Understanding these circumstances will help you recognize when a relationship is beyond repair and when maintaining it poses more harm than benefit.

Recognizing the signs that indicate it's time to sever ties is crucial for making an informed decision. These signs can include repeated patterns of abuse, consistent feelings of fear or anxiety around the family member, and significant negative impacts on your mental health. We will provide you with tools to identify these red flags and help you assess the health of your relationships objectively.

Red Flags in Toxic Family Relationships

The following are warning signs you may need to walk away from an unhealthy family member:

- You feel insecure.
- You feel unloved.
- You feel unsafe.
- You do not feel valued.
- You do not trust the family member.
- The family member is abusing you or is domestically violent. (Take immediate action if you are in an abusive or violent home.)
- The family member blames you for everything wrong with the relationship.
- The family member blames you for their weaknesses and problems.
- The family member controls your finances or treats you like a servant.
- The family member disrespects and violates your privacy.
- The family member does not accept you unconditionally and points out all the ways you need to change.
- The family member does not accept your authentic self or creates an environment where you are not free to be who you are.
- The family member does not accept your sexual orientation or gender identity.
- The family member has demonstrated their inability or unwillingness to change their harmful behavior.
- The family member is gaslighting you by telling you your interpretation of what is happening is untrue, or you are overreacting.
- The family member isolates you from support systems such as family, friends, church, or employment.

- The family member is manipulating and controlling you.
- The family member is unreliable and keeps breaking promises in ways that hurt you.
- The family member uses religion or Bible verses to shame, manipulate, control, or justify abuse and mistreatment.
- The family member struggles with addiction in ways that harm you.
- The family member's behavior is resulting in your own struggle with addiction.

Walking away from toxic relationships can lead to profound emotional freedom and personal growth. It allows you to reclaim your life, focus on your own needs and well-being, and create a supportive and loving environment for yourself. This process requires immense courage, self-awareness, and an unwavering commitment to your well-being.

When making such a significant decision, it is crucial to set clear and healthy boundaries, manage feelings of guilt and obligation, and seek support from trusted friends, professionals, and support groups. If you are in danger, prioritize your safety by getting to a safe place immediately and calling 911. Once you are safe, reach out for the help and support you need.

This month's journey is not just about ending toxic relationships but about beginning a new chapter of your life where you prioritize your happiness, health, and personal growth. It's about recognizing your worth, embracing your courage, and taking decisive action to create a life filled with love, respect, and authenticity.

Week 1: Making the Decision to Walk Away

Introduction of Week's Theme

Deciding to walk away from toxic family members is one of the most significant and challenging steps in your healing journey. This decision often comes with a complex mix of emotions, including sadness, guilt, fear, and even relief. Letting go of long-held connections and confronting deeply ingrained family dynamics can be painful, but it is also a crucial step toward reclaiming your life and well-being.

The impact of toxic relationships on your overall well-being cannot be overstated. Toxic family dynamics can lead to chronic stress, anxiety, depression, and other mental health issues. Recognizing the toll these relationships take on your health is a critical step in understanding the necessity of walking away.

Self-awareness and self-reflection are essential in this process. Reflecting on your experiences, emotions, and needs provides clarity and insight into whether continuing the relationship is beneficial for you. Honest introspection about how the relationship affects your sense of self-worth, happiness, and personal growth is vital.

Boundaries play a crucial role in toxic relationships. Setting and maintaining healthy boundaries is essential for protecting yourself from further harm. However, despite your best efforts, toxic family members may continue to violate them. Repeated disregard for boundaries is a strong indicator that it's time to walk away.

Societal and cultural pressures can influence your decision. Many people feel obligated to maintain family relationships due to societal norms or cultural expectations, even when those relationships are harmful. It's important to challenge these pressures and recognize that your well-being is paramount. You are not obligated to maintain relationships that cause you harm.

Feelings of guilt and obligation often accompany the decision to cut ties. Guilt can be a significant barrier to making healthy decisions, as toxic family members may manipulate you into feeling responsible for the relationship's failure. Learning to release this guilt and affirm your right to prioritize your health is a vital part of the process.

Practical exercises can help you assess your relationships, weigh the pros and cons, and visualize the potential benefits of walking away. These exercises will empower you to make a decision that aligns with your values and needs.

Seeking support during this time is crucial. Deciding to cut ties is not something you have to do alone. Friends, therapists, and support groups can provide valuable guidance, encouragement, and validation as you navigate this challenging process.

By understanding the factors to consider when deciding to walk away from toxic family members, you will feel more empowered to make a decision that prioritizes your well-being and sets the stage for a healthier, happier future. This week is about facing difficult truths and making choices that support your healing and personal growth. You deserve to live a life free from toxic influences, where you are valued, respected, and able to thrive.

March 1
- **Affirmation:** "I have the right to protect myself from harm."
- **Reflection:** "Your well-being is a priority, and it is okay to make choices that safeguard your health."
- **Practical Exercise:** Write about a situation where you felt harmed by a family member. Reflect on how protecting yourself can lead to better outcomes.

March 2
- **Affirmation:** "I trust my judgment in making decisions about my relationships."
- **Reflection:** "You know your situation best. Trust yourself to make the right decisions."
- **Practical Exercise:** Make a list of pros and cons regarding continuing a relationship with a toxic family

member. Reflect on your findings.

March 3

- **Affirmation:** "I deserve to be surrounded by supportive and loving people."
- **Reflection:** "Supportive relationships are essential for your well-being."
- **Practical Exercise:** Identify the supportive and loving people in your life. Reflect on how these relationships make you feel.

March 4

- **Affirmation:** "I am not obligated to maintain relationships that harm me."
- **Reflection:** "It is okay to let go of relationships that are detrimental to your health."
- **Practical Exercise:** Reflect on societal or cultural pressures that make you feel obligated to maintain toxic relationships. Write about why it is okay to break free from these pressures.

March 5

- **Affirmation:** "I can let go of the guilt associated with cutting ties."
- **Reflection:** "Guilt can be a significant barrier to making healthy decisions. Release it."
- **Practical Exercise:** Write a letter to yourself, forgiving any guilt you feel about considering cutting ties with a toxic family member.

March 6

- **Affirmation:** "I will consider the long-term effects of my decisions."
- **Reflection:** "Thinking about the long-term impact can help guide your decisions."
- **Practical Exercise:** Write down the potential long-term effects of walking away from a toxic family member on your mental health and future relationships.

March 7

- **Affirmation:** "I will seek professional guidance if needed."
- **Reflection:** "Professional support can provide valuable insights and guidance."
- **Practical Exercise:** Research and list professionals (therapists, counselors) who specialize in family dynamics. Schedule a consultation if needed.

Week 2: Issues to Consider Before Walking Away

Introduction of Week's Theme

Before making the final decision to cut ties with toxic family members, it's crucial to consider a range of factors to ensure that your decision is well-informed and holistic. Walking away from toxic relationships is a significant step that can profoundly impact your life, so it is essential to weigh all aspects carefully.

Consider the impact on your mental and emotional health. Toxic relationships can cause significant psychological harm, leading to chronic stress, anxiety, depression, and other mental health issues. Assess how maintaining these relationships affects your overall well-being and whether severing ties might lead to improved mental health and emotional stability. Reflect on the relief and peace that may come from distancing yourself from harmful interactions.

Think about the implications for other family relationships. Cutting ties with one family member can affect your relationships with others within the family system. It's important to anticipate potential reactions and prepare for how these dynamics might shift. Consider how you will navigate these changes and maintain or strengthen healthy family connections that support your well-being.

Reflect on your future well-being. Consider the long-term benefits of ending toxic relationships, such as the potential for personal growth, freedom from emotional manipulation, and the ability to focus on nurturing positive relationships. Visualize a future where you are free from the constraints of toxicity and able to pursue your goals and dreams without interference.

Financial and practical considerations are also important. Assess your financial independence and stability, especially if you have been reliant on family support. Ensure that you have a solid plan in place to manage your finances and practical needs independently. This might involve securing employment, housing, or other resources to support your transition.

Seek professional guidance if needed. Therapists, counselors, and support groups can provide valuable insights and support as you navigate this challenging decision. Professional guidance can help you process your emotions, develop effective strategies, and ensure that your decision aligns with your overall well-being.

Prepare yourself emotionally and mentally for the potential conflict that might arise from cutting ties. Develop strategies to cope with guilt, anger, or attempts to manipulate you into maintaining the relationship. Having a plan in place can help you stay firm in your decision and protect your emotional health.

As you explore these considerations, know that you are taking important steps toward creating a healthier, more fulfilling life. Your well-being is paramount, and by carefully evaluating these aspects, you are honoring your worth and paving the way for a brighter future. Let's commit to this process with compassion and determination, knowing that the decision to walk away, if made, will be one rooted in self-love and the pursuit of a healthier, happier life.

March 8
  - **Affirmation:** "I will weigh the impact on other family

members."

- **Reflection:** "Consider how your decision will affect other family relationships."
- **Practical Exercise:** Write about the potential impact of your decision on other family members. Reflect on ways to manage these relationships.

March 9

- **Affirmation:** "I will prioritize my mental and emotional health."
- **Reflection:** "Your health should be the main factor in your decision."
- **Practical Exercise:** Reflect on how maintaining the toxic relationship affects your mental and emotional health. Write about the benefits of prioritizing your well-being.

March 10

- **Affirmation:** "I will consider my financial and practical situation."
- **Reflection:** "Practical considerations are important in the decision-making process."
- **Practical Exercise:** Assess your financial and practical situation. Write about how cutting ties might affect these aspects of your life and plan accordingly.

March 11

- **Affirmation:** "I will seek professional guidance to ensure my decision is well-informed."
- **Reflection:** "Professional guidance can provide valuable insights and support."
- **Practical Exercise:** Identify a therapist or counselor you can speak with about your situation. Schedule a consultation to discuss your decision.

March 12

- **Affirmation:** "I will prepare for potential emotional and mental challenges."
- **Reflection:** "Anticipating emotional and mental challenges can help you remain resolute."
- **Practical Exercise:** Write down potential emotional

and mental challenges you might face. Plan strategies to cope with these challenges.

March 13
- **Affirmation:** "I will maintain firm boundaries throughout the process."
- **Reflection:** "Firm boundaries are crucial to protecting yourself."
- **Practical Exercise:** Write down the boundaries you need to maintain during and after the process of cutting ties. Reflect on how you will enforce them.

March 14
- **Affirmation:** "I will take time to heal and recover after ending the relationship."
- **Reflection:** "Healing is a necessary part of moving forward."
- **Practical Exercise:** Create a self-care plan to follow after ending the toxic relationship. Include activities that support your emotional and mental recovery.

Week 3: Warning Signs You May Need to Cut Ties

Introduction of Week's Theme

Recognizing the warning signs that indicate it may be time to cut ties with a toxic family member is crucial for your mental, emotional, and physical well-being. Toxic relationships can be insidious, often masking their harmful effects behind a facade of normalcy or familial obligation. Understanding these warning signs empowers you to make informed and self-affirming decisions about your relationships.

The impact of toxic family dynamics can be profound and far-reaching. Repeated exposure to manipulative behaviors, chronic negativity, and emotional or physical abuse can erode your self-esteem, create chronic stress, and lead to various mental health issues such as anxiety, depression, and PTSD. Recognizing these patterns and understanding their effects on your well-being is the first step toward reclaiming your life and ensuring your safety.

Several critical warning signs may indicate it's time to consider severing ties with a toxic family member:

- **Chronic Boundary Violations:** When a family member consistently disregards your boundaries, it's a clear sign of disrespect and a lack of regard for your well-being. These violations can take many forms, from ignoring your personal space and privacy to dismissing your emotional needs and preferences.
- **Emotional Manipulation:** Manipulative behaviors, such as gaslighting, guilt-tripping, and emotional blackmail, are designed to control and undermine you. These tactics can leave you doubting your perceptions, feeling guilty for asserting your needs, and trapped in a cycle of emotional dependency.
- **Consistent Emotional Drainage:** Feeling consistently drained, anxious, or fearful after interactions with a family member is a significant red flag. Your energy and emotional state are valuable indicators of the health of your relationships. If you find yourself dreading interactions or needing extensive recovery time afterward, it's essential to acknowledge this impact.
- **Deterioration of Mental Health:** Noticeable declines in your mental health, such as increased anxiety, depression, or a sense of hopelessness, can often be traced back to toxic family interactions. Recognizing this connection is vital for taking proactive steps to protect your mental well-being.
- **Physical Symptoms of Stress:** Chronic stress from toxic family dynamics can manifest in physical symptoms such as headaches, insomnia, digestive issues, and other stress-related ailments. These physical indicators are your body's way of signaling that something is wrong and needs to be addressed.
- **Pattern of Abuse or Neglect:** Any form of

abuse—emotional, physical, or psychological—is unacceptable. Similarly, chronic neglect, where your needs and well-being are consistently disregarded, can be equally damaging. Recognizing these patterns is crucial for making decisions that prioritize your safety and health.

- **Isolation from Support Networks:** Toxic family members often try to isolate you from friends, other family members, and support networks. This isolation increases their control over you and reduces your ability to seek help. Recognizing attempts at isolation is vital to maintaining your independence and support systems.

This week is about empowering you with the knowledge and tools to recognize when a relationship is doing more harm than good. It's about validating your experiences and feelings, understanding that it's okay to protect yourself, and taking the necessary steps to create a healthier, more supportive environment for yourself.

Remember that you have the right to prioritize your well-being and safety. Trust your instincts, honor your experiences, and know that recognizing these warning signs is a courageous and crucial step in your healing journey. Gain clarity, strength, and empowerment to make the best decisions for your future.

March 15

- **Affirmation:** "I recognize when my boundaries are consistently violated."
- **Reflection:** "Repeated boundary violations are a significant warning sign."
- **Practical Exercise:** Write about instances when your boundaries were violated. Reflect on the patterns and frequency.

March 16

- **Affirmation:** "I am aware of manipulative behaviors aimed at controlling me."
- **Reflection:** "Manipulation is a common tactic in toxic

relationships."
  - **Practical Exercise:** List manipulative behaviors you have experienced. Reflect on how they make you feel and their impact on your life.

March 17

  - **Affirmation:** "I notice when I feel drained after interactions."
  - **Reflection:** "Feeling consistently drained is a key indicator of a toxic relationship."
  - **Practical Exercise:** Keep a journal of your emotional state before and after interactions with a toxic family member. Reflect on the differences.

March 18

  - **Affirmation:** "I acknowledge when my mental health is deteriorating due to a relationship."
  - **Reflection:** "Your mental health is a crucial indicator of the health of your relationships."
  - **Practical Exercise:** Reflect on changes in your mental health since being involved with the toxic family member. Write about how the relationship contributes to these changes.

March 19

  - **Affirmation:** "I will not ignore physical symptoms of stress caused by toxic interactions."
  - **Reflection:** "Physical symptoms can be a manifestation of emotional stress."
  - **Practical Exercise:** Keep track of physical symptoms you experience during stressful family interactions. Write about the correlation between these symptoms and your interactions.

March 20

  - **Affirmation:** "I recognize patterns of abuse or neglect."
  - **Reflection:** "Any form of abuse or chronic neglect is a clear sign of toxicity."
  - **Practical Exercise:** Write about any patterns of abuse or neglect you have experienced. Reflect on how these patterns have affected you.

March 21

- **Affirmation:** "I deserve to have supportive and respectful relationships."
- **Reflection:** "You have the right to be treated with respect and support."
- **Practical Exercise:** Reflect on attempts by toxic family members to isolate you from your support networks. Write about how you can strengthen these supportive relationships.

Week 4: How to Cut Ties with Toxic Family Members

Introduction of Week's Theme

Deciding to cut ties with toxic family members is a significant step that requires careful planning, support, and emotional fortitude. Implementing this decision involves creating a clear and detailed plan for ending the toxic relationship. A structured approach can help you navigate the complexities and emotional turbulence that may arise, including what you will say, how you will communicate your decision, and strategies for handling potential responses from toxic family members.

Support is crucial during this time. Identifying and seeking out trusted friends, professionals, and support groups can offer guidance, understanding, and encouragement. These individuals provide a much-needed buffer and source of strength as you go through the difficult process of cutting ties.

Maintaining firm boundaries is another critical aspect. Establishing and enforcing these boundaries during and after the separation process protects your emotional and mental health, ensuring that you can move forward without being drawn back into toxic dynamics.

Preparation for potential backlash is essential. Toxic family members may react with anger, guilt-tripping, or attempts to re-establish control. Strategies to prepare for these reactions can help you remain resolute and firm in your decision despite any negative responses.

Healing and recovery after ending a toxic relationship are vital. Creating a self-care plan that includes activities and practices to support your emotional and mental recovery is necessary to rebuild your sense of self and cultivate a life free from toxic influences.

This challenging process is a crucial step toward creating a life where you are free to thrive, unburdened by the harmful dynamics of toxic relationships. Embrace this opportunity to take decisive action for your health and happiness, knowing that each step you take is a powerful affirmation of your worth and your right to a peaceful, respectful, and fulfilling life.

March 22
- **Affirmation:** "I will create a clear plan to end the toxic relationship."
- **Reflection:** "Having a plan helps make the process smoother and less stressful."
- **Practical Exercise:** Outline a clear plan for ending the toxic relationship, including what you will say and how you will handle potential responses.

March 23
- **Affirmation:** "I will ensure my safety and well-being during the process."
- **Reflection:** "Your safety is paramount. Take necessary precautions."
- **Practical Exercise:** Identify steps you can take to ensure your safety, such as changing locks, updating security systems, or seeking a safe place to stay if needed.

March 24
- **Affirmation:** "I will document important interactions to protect myself."

- **Reflection:** "Documentation can provide evidence and clarity if conflicts arise."
- **Practical Exercise:** Start a journal or file where you record significant interactions with the toxic family member, including dates, times, and details of conversations or incidents.

March 25

- **Affirmation:** "I will communicate my decision clearly and calmly."
- **Reflection:** "Clear communication helps avoid misunderstandings."
- **Practical Exercise:** Write a script for how you will communicate your decision to the toxic family member. Practice delivering it calmly and confidently.

March 26

- **Affirmation:** "I will seek support from trusted friends and professionals."
- **Reflection:** "Support is essential when making significant life changes."
- **Practical Exercise:** Identify at least two people you can rely on for support during this process. Reach out to them and discuss your plan.

March 27

- **Affirmation:** "I will create a supportive environment for my healing."
- **Reflection:** "A supportive environment is crucial for recovery and growth."
- **Practical Exercise:** Identify elements that contribute to a supportive environment. Make changes in your living space to enhance comfort and positivity.

March 28

- **Affirmation:** "I will engage in activities that bring me joy and peace."
- **Reflection:** "Joyful activities can aid in emotional recovery."
- **Practical Exercise:** Make a list of activities that bring you joy and peace. Commit to engaging in at least one

of these activities each day.

March 29

- **Affirmation:** "I will reconnect with my passions and interests."
- **Reflection:** "Reconnecting with passions can restore a sense of self."
- **Practical Exercise:** Identify a passion or interest you have neglected. Plan a specific time to engage in this activity and reflect on the experience.

March 30

- **Affirmation:** "I am reclaiming my life and my happiness."
- **Reflection:** "Cutting ties with a toxic family member is a step towards reclaiming your life."
- **Practical Exercise:** Reflect on the positive changes you anticipate in your life after ending the toxic relationship. Write them down as a source of motivation.

March 31

- **Affirmation:** "I am empowered to create a healthy and fulfilling future."
- **Reflection:** "Empowerment comes from taking control of your life and decisions."
- **Practical Exercise:** Visualize your future free from toxic influences. Create a vision board or write a detailed description of what your healthy, fulfilling future looks like.

March Conclusion

As we conclude this month's focus on when to cut ties and walk away from toxic family members, take a moment to reflect deeply on the knowledge and insights you have gained. This month's journey has been challenging, but it has also been a powerful step toward reclaiming your life and prioritizing your mental and emotional well-being. Deciding to end a toxic relationship is never easy, but it is a crucial step toward creating a healthier, more fulfilling life.

Remember, you have the right to prioritize your health and happiness. Trust your judgment, seek support, and stay committed to your journey of healing. Each step you take toward creating a healthier environment for yourself is a testament to your courage and resilience.

Important Principles to Remember When Walking Away

As you move forward on your healing journey and make the decision whether or not to walk away from toxic family dynamics, keep these important principles in mind:

- **Decision-Making:** Weigh the pros and cons and make informed decisions about your relationships. This skill empowers you to take control of your life and make choices that align with your best interests.
- **Boundary Setting:** Practice setting and maintaining boundaries to protect your well-being. Boundaries are essential for safeguarding your mental and emotional health and ensuring that you are treated with respect and dignity.
- **Self-Compassion:** Cultivate self-compassion, allowing yourself to release guilt and prioritize your health. Self-compassion helps you to be kind to yourself, especially during difficult times, and reinforces your worthiness of love and care.
- **Support Seeking:** Identify and seek support from trusted friends and professionals. Recognizing the importance of a support system is crucial for navigating challenging decisions and finding strength in the encouragement and understanding of others.
- **Courage and Resilience:** Recognize and celebrate your courage and resilience in facing and making difficult decisions. Your bravery in confronting toxic dynamics and your ability to persevere through adversity are commendable and inspire continued growth.

Celebrate your progress and acknowledge the strength you have demonstrated throughout this month. Each boundary set, each moment of self-compassion, and each step taken toward severing toxic ties is a victory. These accomplishments are significant milestones on your journey to recovery and personal growth.

Keep trusting in your journey. Embrace the uncertainty with confidence, knowing that you have the strength and resilience to overcome any challenge. You are building a life that is aligned with your true self, a life that honors your values and passions. Each day is an opportunity to reaffirm your commitment to yourself and to take another step toward healing.

April: Boundaries and Healthy Relationships

Establishing and maintaining healthy boundaries is essential for creating relationships that are respectful, supportive, and fulfilling. Boundaries let others know where they stop and you start. Boundaries serve as the invisible lines that define your personal limits and protect your well-being. They foster mutual respect, create a sense of safety in interactions, and ensure that your needs and values are honored. This month, we will focus on understanding the critical importance of boundaries, how to set them effectively, and how to nurture and maintain healthy relationships that respect these boundaries.

Healthy boundaries are vital for protecting your mental, emotional, and physical well-being. They help you manage your relationships by clearly defining what is acceptable and what is not. Without boundaries, relationships can become unbalanced, leading to feelings of resentment, stress, and burnout. By learning to communicate your needs clearly and assertively, you can build stronger, more positive relationships that contribute to your overall happiness and mental health.

This month's journey is about more than just learning to say "no" to people regarding their actions and behavior. It's about creating a life where your values and needs are respected, where you feel safe and supported, and where your relationships are balanced and fulfilling.

Week 1: Setting Healthy Boundaries

Introduction of Week's Theme

Setting healthy boundaries is a fundamental aspect of maintaining your well-being and ensuring your relationships are respectful and fulfilling. Boundaries help you protect your personal space, emotions, and time. This week, we will explore the basics of boundary-setting, focusing on how to recognize your limits, communicate them effectively, and enforce them with confidence and compassion.

Understanding your personal limits is the first step in establishing healthy boundaries. It involves introspection and self-awareness, allowing you to identify what makes you feel comfortable, respected, and safe. These limits can vary in different contexts and relationships, making it essential to tailor your boundaries to suit your unique needs and situations. We will explore techniques to help you gain clarity on your personal limits and understand why they are crucial for your mental and emotional health.

Once you have identified your limits, the next step is to communicate them clearly and assertively. Effective communication is critical to ensuring that others understand and respect your boundaries. This involves using clear and concise language, maintaining a calm and respectful tone, and being consistent in your messaging. We will practice crafting boundary statements and role-playing scenarios to build your confidence in articulating your needs.

Maintaining boundaries can sometimes be challenging, especially if you are not used to asserting yourself or if you face resistance from others. It is important to stand firm in your boundaries, even if it feels uncomfortable at first. Consistency and persistence are vital in reinforcing your limits and ensuring that they are respected over time.

April 1
- **Affirmation:** "I have the right to set boundaries that protect my well-being."
- **Reflection:** "Your well-being is a priority, and setting boundaries is a key part of protecting it."
- **Practical Exercise:** Identify an area of your life where you need stronger boundaries. Write down specific boundaries you can set to protect your well-being.

April 2
- **Affirmation:** "I can communicate my boundaries clearly and respectfully."
- **Reflection:** "Clear communication is essential for setting effective boundaries."
- **Practical Exercise:** Practice stating your boundaries in a clear and respectful manner. Role-play with a friend or in front of a mirror.

April 3
- **Affirmation:** "I will stand firm in my boundaries, even if it feels uncomfortable."
- **Reflection:** "Standing firm in your boundaries is a crucial part of maintaining them."
- **Practical Exercise:** Reflect on a situation where you struggled to maintain your boundaries. Write about how you can stand firm in similar situations in the future.

April 4
- **Affirmation:** "I deserve relationships that respect my boundaries."
- **Reflection:** "Respecting your boundaries is a sign of a healthy relationship."
- **Practical Exercise:** Evaluate your current relationships. Identify which ones respect your boundaries and which ones do not. Reflect on how you can address this imbalance.

April 5

- **Affirmation:** "I can say no without feeling guilty."
- **Reflection:** "Saying no is a valid and necessary part of setting boundaries."
- **Practical Exercise:** Practice saying no in a safe environment. Reflect on any feelings of guilt and remind yourself why it's important to set this boundary.

April 6

- **Affirmation:** "I will enforce my boundaries with kindness and firmness."
- **Reflection:** "Boundaries are most effective when enforced with both kindness and firmness."
- **Practical Exercise:** Write down a recent instance where you struggled to enforce a boundary. Reflect on how you can approach it with kindness and firmness in the future.

April 7

- **Affirmation:** "I will honor my boundaries as a form of self-respect."
- **Reflection:** "Honoring your boundaries is an act of self-respect and self-care."
- **Practical Exercise:** Reflect on how honoring your boundaries has positively impacted your life. Write about the changes you have noticed.

Week 2 Types of Healthy Boundaries

Introduction of Week's Theme

Boundaries come in various forms, each serving a unique and essential function in protecting your well-being and fostering healthy relationships. Understanding these different types of boundaries is crucial because they help you define and maintain your personal limits across various aspects of your life. This week, we will explore the various types of boundaries—physical, emotional, mental, and time—and explore how to set and maintain them effectively to create a balanced and fulfilling life.

Physical Boundaries: Physical boundaries pertain to your personal space and physical well-being. These boundaries help you feel safe and comfortable in your environment. They include your preferences for personal space, touch, and physical proximity. Understanding and respecting physical boundaries is essential for maintaining a sense of safety and comfort in your interactions.

Emotional Boundaries: Emotional boundaries involve your feelings and emotional well-being. They protect your ability to feel and express your emotions without being overwhelmed by others' emotional states. Emotional boundaries help you maintain a healthy emotional state by preventing emotional manipulation and ensuring that you do not take on others' emotional burdens.

Mental Boundaries: Mental boundaries relate to your thoughts, beliefs, and intellectual space. They help you maintain clarity and focus by protecting your right to have your own opinions and thoughts. Mental boundaries are crucial for preserving your cognitive health and preventing mental exhaustion caused by constant debates or arguments over your beliefs.

Time Boundaries: Time boundaries involve how you allocate your time and energy. They help you manage your commitments and prioritize activities that align with your values and goals. Setting time boundaries ensures that you have enough time for self-care, personal interests, and meaningful relationships without feeling overwhelmed or overcommitted.

Setting and maintaining boundaries is an ongoing process that requires self-awareness, assertiveness, and commitment. Embrace this week as an opportunity to deepen your understanding of boundaries and enhance your ability to protect your well-being and foster healthier, more respectful relationships.

April 8

- **Affirmation:** "I will set physical boundaries to protect my personal space."
- **Reflection:** "Physical boundaries help you feel safe and comfortable in your environment."
- **Practical Exercise:** An example of a physical space boundary statement might be: "I need personal space right now, please give me some room." Identify situations where your physical boundaries are often challenged. Plan how you will assert these boundaries in the future.

April 9

- **Affirmation:** "I will establish emotional boundaries to protect my feelings."
- **Reflection:** "Emotional boundaries are essential for maintaining your mental health."
- **Practical Exercise:** An example of an emotional boundary statement might be: "I need to take some time for myself right now to process my feelings." Reflect on a time when your emotional boundaries were crossed. Write about how you can better protect these boundaries moving forward.

April 10

- **Affirmation:** "I can create mental boundaries to protect my thoughts and beliefs."
- **Reflection:** "Mental boundaries help you maintain clarity and focus."
- **Practical Exercise:** An example of a mental boundary statement might be: "I choose not to engage in conversations that negatively impact my peace of mind." Identify areas where you need mental boundaries, such as during discussions or while consuming media. Plan how you will enforce these boundaries.

April 11

- **Affirmation:** "I will respect my time by setting clear boundaries around my schedule."

- **Reflection:** "Time boundaries help you prioritize and manage your commitments effectively."
- **Practical Exercise:** An example of a time boundary statement you might use with a toxic family member is: "I am only available to talk for 30 minutes." Identify relationships where you need stronger time boundaries. Create a plan to protect your time and stick to it.

April 12

- **Affirmation:** "I deserve to have my boundaries respected by others."
- **Reflection:** "Respecting your boundaries is a sign of respect and consideration."
- **Practical Exercise:** Reflect on how others respond to your boundaries. Write about how you can communicate your boundaries more effectively if they are not being respected.

April 13

- **Affirmation:** "I will ensure my boundaries are flexible but firm when necessary."
- **Reflection:** "Flexibility in boundaries allows for adaptation, but firmness ensures they are respected."
- **Practical Exercise:** Reflect on a situation where you had to adapt your boundaries. Write about how you balanced flexibility with firmness.

April 14

- **Affirmation:** "I am committed to maintaining my boundaries for my well-being."
- **Reflection:** "Consistency in maintaining boundaries is crucial for their effectiveness."
- **Practical Exercise:** Identify any challenges you face in maintaining your boundaries consistently. Develop strategies to overcome these challenges.

Week 3: Strong Boundary Statements

Introduction of Week's Theme

Creating strong boundary statements is an essential skill for maintaining healthy relationships and protecting one's well-being. Boundary statements clearly articulate one's limits and expectations, ensuring that others understand and respect one's needs. This week, we will explore the process of crafting these statements, focusing on how to communicate one's boundaries in a way that is both firm and respectful.

Here are several critical aspects of strong boundary statements:

- **Clarity and Precision:** Effective boundary statements are clear and specific. We will explore how to articulate your boundaries in a way that leaves no room for misunderstanding, ensuring that your expectations are communicated precisely.
- **Using "I" Statements:** "I" statements are a powerful tool in boundary-setting, allowing you to express your needs and feelings without blaming or accusing others. We will practice converting traditional boundary statements into "I" statements to enhance their effectiveness and foster better communication.
- **Assertiveness without Aggression:** It's crucial to express your boundaries assertively without crossing the line into aggression. We will work on maintaining a calm and composed demeanor while firmly stating your boundaries, ensuring that you are taken seriously without escalating conflicts.
- **Reaffirming Boundaries:** Sometimes, boundaries need to be reiterated to ensure they are respected over time. We will discuss strategies for reaffirming your boundaries when necessary, helping you to maintain them consistently.
- **Handling Resistance:** Not everyone will immediately respect your boundaries, and you may face resistance. We will explore ways to handle pushback with confidence and poise, ensuring that you stand firm in

your needs without being swayed by others' reactions.

- **Empathy and Respect:** While setting boundaries, it's important to remain empathetic and respectful toward others. We will practice balancing firmness with empathy, fostering healthier and more respectful interactions.

Strong boundary statements are the backbone of effective boundary-setting. They help you to assertively express what you need without resorting to aggression or passivity. By mastering this skill, you will be better equipped to manage interactions with family, friends, colleagues, and even strangers, ensuring that your boundaries are consistently honored.

April 15

- **Affirmation:** "I can articulate my boundaries clearly and confidently."
- **Reflection:** "Clear articulation of your boundaries ensures that others understand and respect them."
- **Practical Exercise:** Write down a boundary statement for a specific situation. Practice saying it out loud confidently.

April 16

- **Affirmation:** "I will use 'I' statements to express my boundaries."
- **Reflection:** "'I' statements help you communicate your boundaries without blaming others."
- **Practical Exercise:** Practice converting a boundary statement into an 'I' statement. For example, "You need to stop interrupting me" becomes "I need to speak without interruptions."

April 17

- **Affirmation:** "I can enforce my boundaries with calm and assertiveness."
- **Reflection:** "Calm assertiveness is key to maintaining your boundaries without escalating conflict."
- **Practical Exercise:** Role-play enforcing a boundary

with calm assertiveness. Reflect on how this approach feels and its effectiveness.

April 18

- **Affirmation:** "I will reaffirm my boundaries as needed."
- **Reflection:** "Reaffirming your boundaries ensures they are respected over time."
- **Practical Exercise:** Identify a situation where you need to reaffirm your boundaries. Plan how you will do this and practice your approach.

April 19

- **Affirmation:** "I deserve to have my boundaries respected without question."
- **Reflection:** "Your boundaries are valid and should be respected without needing justification."
- **Practical Exercise:** Write a boundary statement that you have found difficult to enforce. Reflect on why it is important and how you will reaffirm it.

April 20

- **Affirmation:** "I will communicate my boundaries with empathy."
- **Reflection:** "Communicating with empathy helps maintain respect and understanding."
- **Practical Exercise:** Practice delivering a boundary statement with empathy. Reflect on how it impacts the conversation and the other person's response.

April 21

- **Affirmation:** "I will stand by my boundaries even in the face of resistance."
- **Reflection:** "Standing by your boundaries is essential, even when others resist."
- **Practical Exercise:** Reflect on a time when your boundaries were met with resistance. Write about how you can stay firm in similar situations in the future.

Week 4: Removing Toxic People from Your Inner Circle

Introduction of Week's Theme

Sometimes, setting and maintaining healthy boundaries involves the difficult yet necessary step of removing toxic people from your inner circle to protect your well-being. This process requires a clear understanding of what constitutes a toxic relationship and the courage to take decisive action. Toxic relationships are characterized by consistent patterns of disrespect, manipulation, emotional abuse, and boundary violations. These relationships can drain your energy, undermine your self-esteem, and impede your personal growth.

Identifying toxic relationships is the first step. Signs include consistent negativity, lack of support, emotional manipulation, and persistent boundary violations. Recognizing these patterns helps you understand the necessity of distancing yourself from such influences. Emotional challenges such as guilt, fear, or uncertainty are common when severing ties with toxic individuals. These feelings can stem from long-standing attachments, familial obligations, or societal expectations. It's important to acknowledge these emotions and understand that prioritizing your well-being is not an act of selfishness but an essential step toward a healthier and happier life.

Practical strategies for distancing yourself from toxic relationships include setting clear and firm boundaries, reducing or eliminating contact, and seeking support from trusted friends, family members, or professionals. By taking these steps, you create a more supportive and nurturing environment that fosters your personal growth and well-being. Surrounding yourself with positive influences is equally important. Building a supportive network of friends and loved ones who respect your boundaries and uplift you is crucial for your mental and emotional health. Positive relationships provide the encouragement, love, and validation needed to thrive.

The long-term benefits of removing toxic people from your life include increased self-esteem, improved mental health, and greater emotional freedom. By removing negative influences, you make room for positive relationships that enhance your life and contribute to your overall happiness. Commit to the courageous and empowering journey of removing toxic people from your inner circle. Embrace the tools and strategies provided to protect your well-being and build a supportive network. Remember, you deserve relationships that respect your boundaries and contribute positively to your life. Let's take this step together toward a healthier, more fulfilling future.

April 22

- **Affirmation:** "I have the right to distance myself from toxic relationships."
- **Reflection:** "Distancing yourself from toxic relationships is an act of self-care."
- **Practical Exercise:** Reflect on a toxic relationship in your life. Write about the steps you need to take to distance yourself from this person.

April 23

- **Affirmation:** "I will surround myself with people who uplift and support me."
- **Reflection:** "Positive relationships are crucial for your mental and emotional health."
- **Practical Exercise:** Identify supportive people in your life. Plan how you can spend more time with them and reduce time with toxic individuals.

April 24

- **Affirmation:** "I deserve to have relationships that respect my boundaries and values."
- **Reflection:** "Healthy relationships are based on mutual respect and shared values."
- **Practical Exercise:** Reflect on your core values and how they align with your current relationships. Identify any misalignments and plan how to address them.

April 25

- **Affirmation:** "I will take action to protect myself from toxic influences."
- **Reflection:** "Taking action to protect yourself is a powerful step toward healthier relationships."
- **Practical Exercise:** Write down specific actions you can take to protect yourself from a toxic influence in your life.

April 26

- **Affirmation:** "I am not responsible for the reactions of toxic people."
- **Reflection:** "You are responsible for your actions, not the reactions of others."
- **Practical Exercise:** Reflect on how the fear of others' reactions has impacted your boundary-setting. Write about how you can shift this mindset.

April 27

- **Affirmation:** "I will prioritize my well-being over others' expectations."
- **Reflection:** "Your well-being is more important than conforming to others' expectations."
- **Practical Exercise:** Reflect on a time when you prioritized others' expectations over your well-being. Write about how you can prioritize yourself moving forward.

April 28

- **Affirmation:** "I will seek relationships that nurture and support me."
- **Reflection:** "Nurturing and supportive relationships are essential for your well-being."
- **Practical Exercise:** Identify qualities of relationships that nurture and support you. Reflect on how you can cultivate more of these relationships in your life.

April 29

- **Affirmation:** "I will practice forgiveness but also maintain my boundaries."

- **Reflection:** "Forgiveness is important, but it doesn't mean you should tolerate harmful behavior."
- **Practical Exercise:** Reflect on someone you need to forgive. Write about how you can forgive them while still maintaining your boundaries.

April 30
- **Affirmation:** "I am committed to building healthy and fulfilling relationships."
- **Reflection:** "Commitment to healthy relationships is key to their success."
- **Practical Exercise:** Write a commitment statement to yourself about the type of relationships you want to build. Reflect on the steps you will take to achieve this.

April Conclusion

As we conclude this month's focus on boundaries and healthy relationships, take a moment to reflect on the significant progress you have made in understanding and setting boundaries and nurturing healthier connections. Setting and maintaining boundaries is a continuous process that requires self-awareness, assertiveness, and commitment.

Throughout this month, you have explored various aspects of boundary-setting and healthy relationships. From recognizing your limits and communicating them effectively to identifying and distancing yourself from toxic influences, you have developed a robust toolkit of strategies to protect your well-being and foster positive relationships.

Reflect on the Skills You Have Acquired This Month:

- **Boundary Setting**: You have learned to recognize your limits and communicate them effectively, understanding that your well-being is a priority. You have practiced setting boundaries in different areas of your life, such as physical, emotional, mental, and time boundaries.

- **Types of Boundaries**: You have explored different types of boundaries and how to apply them in various aspects of your life, ensuring that you protect your personal space, feelings, thoughts, and time.
- **Boundary Statements**: You have practiced crafting strong boundary statements and enforcing them with confidence. Using 'I' statements and maintaining calm assertiveness, you have learned to communicate your needs clearly and effectively.
- **Removing Toxic Influences**: You have identified toxic relationships and taken steps to distance yourself from harmful influences. By recognizing the signs of toxic behavior and understanding the impact on your well-being, you have taken decisive action to protect yourself.
- **Healthy Relationship Patterns**: You have worked on breaking unhealthy relationship patterns and fostering positive, supportive connections. By seeking relationships based on mutual respect, open communication, and shared values, you have laid the foundation for a healthier social environment.

Remember, healthy relationships are built on mutual respect, understanding, and clear communication. By practicing the strategies and exercises learned this month, you are taking significant steps toward creating a supportive and fulfilling social environment.

Celebrate your progress, acknowledge your strength, and continue to prioritize your well-being. You have the power to build relationships that honor your boundaries and contribute positively to your life. Keep moving forward with confidence and self-compassion, knowing that each step brings you closer to the healthy relationships you deserve.

May: Self-Care and Recovery

Self-care and recovery are crucial components of healing from the impacts of toxic relationships and environments. This month, we will focus on understanding the importance of self-care, developing a balanced self-care plan, and exploring various recovery techniques that promote mental and emotional well-being.

The journey of self-care involves acknowledging and addressing the neglect and emotional abuse you may have experienced. Laying the foundation with self-care basics is essential, emphasizing the need to prioritize your own well-being and integrating nurturing practices into your daily routine. This includes listening to your body's needs, practicing self-compassion, and forgiving yourself for any lapses in self-care.

Creating a balanced self-care plan that addresses physical, emotional, mental, and spiritual needs is the next step. Through practical exercises such as body scan meditations, emotion journals, and physical activities, you will learn to nurture every aspect of your being. This holistic approach ensures that all areas of your well-being are supported, helping you build a strong foundation for recovery.

Journaling is an effective tool for self-reflection, healing, and personal growth. You will explore different journaling techniques, set goals, track your progress, and use prompts to gain deeper insights into your life.

Meditation techniques promote relaxation, mindfulness, and

emotional balance. From guided meditations to mindfulness practices, you will discover methods to calm your mind and connect with your inner self.

Additional self-care practices such as gratitude, creativity, connecting with nature, deep breathing, prioritizing sleep, seeking support, and practicing self-compassion will be explored. These activities will provide you with a diverse set of tools to support your recovery and overall well-being.

By the end of this month, you will have a thorough understanding of self-care and its vital role in your healing journey. You will have practical tools and routines in place to support your ongoing recovery and personal growth. Remember, self-care is a continuous journey that requires dedication and commitment, but it is essential for your overall well-being. Let's embark on this path together, embracing the transformative power of self-care as we work toward healing from past neglect and emotional wounds.

Week 1: Self-Care After Neglect

Introduction of Week's Theme

Self-care is especially important after experiencing neglect or emotional abuse from toxic family members. These experiences can deeply affect your sense of self-worth, often leading you to neglect your own needs as a survival mechanism. This week, we will focus on rebuilding your self-esteem and integrating nurturing practices into your daily routine to aid in your recovery.

Recognizing the importance of self-care and affirming that you deserve to prioritize your own needs is crucial for laying the groundwork for your healing journey. Understanding that you are worthy of love and care helps you reconnect with your sense of self and begin the process of healing from past wounds.

We will explore practical self-care activities that encourage you to listen to your body, respond with kindness, and develop a consistent self-care routine.

We will introduce practices such as gratitude, which helps shift your focus to the positive aspects of your life and enhances your emotional well-being. Deep breathing exercises will be incorporated as a simple yet effective method to manage stress and promote relaxation.

Throughout the week, you will engage in activities designed to nurture your mind, body, and spirit. From creating personalized self-care routines to writing letters of appreciation to yourself, these exercises aim to foster a compassionate relationship with yourself and support your recovery.

Forgiveness is another key component of this week's theme. We will address the importance of forgiving yourself for any lapses in self-care, understanding that self-compassion and growth are integral parts of the healing process.

By the end of this week, you will have established a foundation of self-care practices that support your overall well-being. You will have learned to recognize and honor your needs, creating a nurturing environment that fosters healing and personal growth. Remember, self-care is a journey, and each step you take brings you closer to a healthier and more fulfilling life. Let's embark on this path together, embracing the transformative power of self-care as we work toward healing from past neglect and emotional wounds.

May 1
- **Affirmation:** "I deserve to take care of myself and prioritize my needs."
- **Reflection:** "Self-care is a vital part of recovery and self-respect."
- **Practical Exercise:** List five self-care activities you enjoy. Commit to doing at least one of these activities

today.

May 2

- **Affirmation:** "I will listen to my body's needs and respond with kindness."
- **Reflection:** "Your body communicates its needs to you. Listening and responding kindly is essential."
- **Practical Exercise:** Practice a body scan meditation to check in with your physical state. Note any areas of tension or discomfort and address them with a self-care activity.

May 3

- **Affirmation:** "I am worthy of love, care, and attention."
- **Reflection:** "You are deserving of the love and care you give to others."
- **Practical Exercise:** Write a letter to yourself expressing love and appreciation. Read it aloud and reflect on how it makes you feel.

May 4

- **Affirmation:** "I will create a daily self-care routine that supports my well-being."
- **Reflection:** "A consistent self-care routine helps maintain your mental and emotional health."
- **Practical Exercise:** Design a daily self-care routine that includes activities for your mind, body, and spirit. Implement it today.

May 5

- **Affirmation:** "I will forgive myself for any lapses in self-care."
- **Reflection:** "Forgiveness is a key part of self-compassion and growth."
- **Practical Exercise:** Reflect on times when you neglected self-care. Write about how you can forgive yourself and commit to improving.

May 6

- **Affirmation:** "I will practice gratitude to enhance my emotional well-being."

- **Reflection:** "Gratitude helps shift your focus to the positive aspects of your life."
- **Practical Exercise:** Write a daily gratitude list, noting at least three things you are grateful for each day. Reflect on how this practice affects your mood and perspective.

May 7

- **Affirmation:** "I will practice deep breathing to reduce stress and promote relaxation."
- **Reflection:** "Deep breathing is a simple yet effective tool for managing stress."
- **Practical Exercise:** Practice deep breathing exercises for five minutes. Reflect on the impact this has on your stress levels and sense of calm.

Week 2: Balanced Self-Care Plan

Introduction of Week's Theme

Creating a balanced self-care plan involves addressing various aspects of your life and ensuring that your physical, emotional, mental, and spiritual needs are all nurtured. This week, we will explore the components of a healing self-care plan that supports your overall well-being and promotes sustained recovery.

A balanced self-care plan starts with understanding that your well-being is multifaceted. It's not enough to focus on just one area; all aspects of your life are interconnected. We will explore how to create harmony among these different aspects, allowing you to develop a holistic approach to self-care.

Balancing your self-care activities to nurture your whole self involves identifying and integrating practices that support your physical health. Engaging in enjoyable physical activities strengthens your body and improves your energy levels.

Emotional self-care is vital, recognizing the importance of acknowledging and expressing your feelings. Emotional well-being is essential for mental health, and by starting an emotion journal, you can provide yourself with a safe space to explore and process your emotions.

Mental self-care will also be a key focus, as stimulating and calming your mind is crucial for overall health. Activities that challenge and relax your mind, such as reading or solving puzzles, can help maintain mental sharpness and reduce stress.

Spiritual self-care connects you to your inner self and brings a sense of peace and joy. You will explore spiritual practices that resonate with you, whether it's meditation, nature walks, or prayer. These activities help nourish your spirit and provide a deeper sense of fulfillment.

We will emphasize the importance of self-compassion and gentleness with yourself. Writing a self-compassionate letter and engaging in activities that bring you joy and fulfillment are crucial steps in building a sustainable self-care routine. By being kind to yourself and prioritizing your needs, you foster a supportive environment for healing and growth.

Each day will provide affirmations, reflections, and practical exercises to help you integrate these practices into your life. By the end of the week, you will have a well-rounded self-care plan that addresses all aspects of your well-being. This balanced approach will not only support your recovery but also enhance your overall happiness and quality of life. Let's take this journey together, focusing on holistic self-care and nurturing every part of who you are.

May 8
- **Affirmation:** "I will balance my self-care activities to nurture my whole self."
- **Reflection:** "A balanced approach to self-care ensures all areas of your well-being are addressed."
- **Practical Exercise:** Create a self-care wheel divided into sections (physical, emotional, mental, spiritual). Write

self-care activities for each section and commit to practicing them.

May 9

- **Affirmation:** "I will include physical activities in my self-care plan to strengthen my body."
- **Reflection:** "Physical self-care is essential for maintaining your health and energy levels."
- **Practical Exercise:** Choose a physical activity you enjoy (e.g., walking, yoga, dancing). Incorporate it into your routine this week.

May 10

- **Affirmation:** "I will practice emotional self-care by acknowledging and expressing my feelings."
- **Reflection:** "Emotional self-care involves recognizing and honoring your emotions."
- **Practical Exercise:** Start an emotion journal. Write about your feelings each day and reflect on how you can support yourself emotionally.

May 11

- **Affirmation:** "I will engage in mental self-care to stimulate and calm my mind."
- **Reflection:** "Mental self-care includes activities that challenge and relax your mind."
- **Practical Exercise:** Choose a mental self-care activity (e.g., reading, puzzles, meditation). Dedicate time to it today and reflect on its impact.

May 12

- **Affirmation:** "I will nurture my spirit through practices that bring me peace and joy."
- **Reflection:** "Spiritual self-care connects you to your inner self and brings a sense of peace."
- **Practical Exercise:** Engage in a spiritual self-care practice (e.g., meditation, nature walks, prayer). Reflect on how it nourishes your spirit.

May 13

- **Affirmation:** "I will practice self-compassion and be

gentle with myself."
  - **Reflection:** "Self-compassion is crucial for healing and growth."
  - **Practical Exercise:** Write a self-compassionate letter to yourself, acknowledging your struggles and offering kindness and support. Reflect on how this exercise makes you feel.

May 14
  - **Affirmation:** "I will engage in activities that bring me joy and fulfillment."
  - **Reflection:** "Pursuing activities you love enhances your overall happiness."
  - **Practical Exercise:** Identify an activity that brings you joy and fulfillment. Dedicate time to this activity and reflect on its impact on your mood and sense of satisfaction.

Week 3: How to Journal

Introduction of Week's Theme

Journaling is a powerful tool for self-reflection, healing, and personal growth. By exploring different journaling techniques, you can support your recovery and self-care journey effectively.

Journaling provides a safe space to explore your thoughts and emotions, serving as a healthy outlet for self-expression. It allows you to delve into your inner world, gain insights into your feelings, and track your progress over time. Regularly writing about your experiences creates a written record that can reveal patterns, highlight growth, and provide clarity.

The basics of daily journaling involve writing about your thoughts, feelings, and experiences each day. This practice helps you stay connected to your emotional landscape and fosters a habit of self-reflection. Consistency in journaling enhances your ability to understand and process your emotions.

Using journaling as a tool for goal setting and tracking progress can be transformative. By articulating your short-term and long-term goals in writing, you develop a clear roadmap for your recovery and personal growth. Tracking your progress helps you stay motivated and recognize the strides you are making, reinforcing your commitment to self-improvement.

Reviewing your journal entries is an essential part of the process. Reflecting on what you have written over time allows you to gain deeper insights, recognize recurring themes, and understand your emotional patterns. This review process is crucial for acknowledging your progress and identifying areas for further growth.

Incorporating journaling into your daily routine can be a supportive tool for your self-care and recovery journey. Through consistent practice, journaling can become a cherished habit that enhances your self-awareness, emotional health, and personal development. Embrace the transformative power of journaling and use it as a means to nurture your mind, body, and spirit.

May 15

- **Affirmation:** "I will use journaling as a tool for self-discovery and healing."
- **Reflection:** "Journaling helps you explore your thoughts and emotions in a safe space."
- **Practical Exercise:** Start a daily journal. Write about your thoughts, feelings, and experiences each day. Reflect on the process and any insights gained.

May 16

- **Affirmation:** "I can express my emotions freely through journaling."
- **Reflection:** "Journaling provides a safe outlet for expressing your emotions."
- **Practical Exercise:** Write a free-form journal entry expressing your emotions without censoring yourself. Reflect on how it feels to release your emotions on paper.

May 17

- **Affirmation:** "I will use journaling to process difficult emotions."
- **Reflection:** "Journaling helps you process and understand complex feelings."
- **Practical Exercise:** Write about a recent experience that brought up difficult emotions. Explore these feelings in detail, allowing yourself to fully express and understand them.

May 18

- **Affirmation:** "I will use journaling to set goals and track my progress."
- **Reflection:** "Setting goals and tracking progress helps you stay focused and motivated."
- **Practical Exercise:** Write about your short-term and long-term goals. Reflect on the steps you need to take to achieve them and track your progress.

May 19

- Affirmation: "I will journal as if I am writing to my closest friend, myself."
- **Reflection:** "Writing to yourself as a friend fosters self-compassion and honesty."
- Practical Exercise: Write a journal entry as if you are confiding in your closest friend, who is yourself. Be open and kind, sharing your thoughts and feelings without judgment. Reflect on how this approach affects your self-perception and emotional state.

May 20

- **Affirmation:** "I will review my journal entries to gain insights and track my growth."
- **Reflection:** "Reviewing your journal entries helps you recognize patterns and progress."
- **Practical Exercise:** Review your journal entries from the past week. Write about any patterns or insights you notice and how they inform your self-care journey.

May 21

- **Affirmation:** "I will practice mindfulness to stay present and connected."
- **Reflection:** "Mindfulness helps you stay grounded and connected to the present moment."
- **Practical Exercise:** Practice a mindfulness exercise, such as mindful eating or walking. Reflect on how staying present affects your thoughts and feelings.

Week 4: How to Meditate

Introduction of Week's Theme

Meditation is a powerful practice that promotes relaxation, mindfulness, and emotional balance. Let's explore different meditation techniques and how they can enhance your self-care and recovery process.

Meditation helps you achieve a state of calm and relaxation by focusing your mind and reducing stress. Guided meditation is a great starting point for beginners. It provides structure and support, making it easier to follow along and experience the benefits. In guided meditation, a narrator will lead you through the process, helping you focus on your breath, body, or specific visualizations.

Mindfulness meditation focuses on staying present in the moment. By concentrating on your breath and bodily sensations, mindfulness meditation helps you cultivate awareness and reduce anxiety. This practice is particularly effective in helping you stay grounded and connected to the present rather than being overwhelmed by past experiences or future worries.

There are various meditation techniques to explore. Loving-kindness meditation involves silently repeating phrases that convey good wishes for yourself and others, promoting compassion and emotional connection. Body scan meditation guides you through paying attention to different parts of your body, promoting relaxation and awareness. Mantra meditation involves silently repeating a word or phrase to help focus your mind and reduce distractions.

Consistency is key in meditation. Making meditation a regular part of your daily routine enhances its benefits over time. Setting aside a specific time each day for meditation can help you integrate this practice into your life, leading to sustained improvements in your mental and emotional well-being.

Meditation also fosters a deeper connection with your inner self. By gaining insights into your thoughts and emotions, meditation promotes self-awareness and personal growth. Creative activities, such as drawing or painting, can also serve as a form of meditation, providing an outlet for self-expression and relaxation. Engaging in these activities mindfully helps you achieve a meditative state, allowing you to focus on the present moment and experience a sense of calm.

Connecting with nature is another form of meditation. Spending time outdoors in a natural setting rejuvenates your mind and body, promoting a sense of peace and well-being. Nature has a calming and restorative effect, helping you feel more grounded and connected to the world around you.

By incorporating these meditation techniques into your routine, you will develop a deeper understanding of how meditation can support your self-care and recovery journey. Embrace these practices and continue to explore and refine your meditation routine, knowing that each step brings you closer to inner peace and emotional balance.

May 22
- **Affirmation:** "I will practice meditation to calm my mind and body."
- **Reflection:** "Meditation helps you achieve a state of calm and relaxation."
- **Practical Exercise:** Practice a guided meditation for

beginners. Reflect on how the practice makes you feel and its impact on your state of mind.

May 23

- **Affirmation:** "I can use mindfulness meditation to stay present in the moment."
- **Reflection:** "Mindfulness meditation helps you focus on the present and reduce stress."
- **Practical Exercise:** Practice mindfulness meditation, focusing on your breathing and sensations. Reflect on how staying present affects your thoughts and feelings.

May 24

- **Affirmation:** "I will explore different meditation techniques to find what works best for me."
- **Reflection:** "Experimenting with various techniques helps you discover what resonates with you."
- **Practical Exercise:** Try a new meditation technique (e.g., loving-kindness, body scan, or mantra meditation). Reflect on how it differs from other methods you've tried.

May 25

- **Affirmation:** "I will make time for regular meditation practice in my daily routine."
- **Reflection:** "Consistent practice enhances the benefits of meditation."
- **Practical Exercise:** Set aside a specific time each day for meditation. Reflect on how making meditation a regular part of your routine affects your well-being.

May 26

- **Affirmation:** "I will use meditation to connect with my inner self and find peace."
- **Reflection:** "Meditation fosters a deeper connection with your inner self."
- **Practical Exercise:** Practice a meditation that focuses on inner peace and self-connection. Reflect on the insights and feelings that arise during the practice.

May 27

- **Affirmation:** "I will engage in creative activities to express myself."
- **Reflection:** "Creative activities provide an outlet for self-expression and relaxation."
- **Practical Exercise:** Choose a creative activity (e.g., drawing, painting, writing, music). Spend time engaging in this activity and reflect on how it makes you feel.

May 28

- **Affirmation:** "I will connect with nature to rejuvenate my mind and body."
- **Reflection:** "Nature has a calming and restorative effect on your well-being."
- **Practical Exercise:** Spend time outdoors in a natural setting. Reflect on how connecting with nature affects your state of mind and physical well-being.

May 29

- **Affirmation:** "I will prioritize sleep to support my overall health."
- **Reflection:** "Adequate sleep is essential for physical and mental health."
- **Practical Exercise:** Establish a bedtime routine that promotes good sleep hygiene. Reflect on how improving your sleep habits affects your overall well-being.

May 30

- **Affirmation:** "I will seek support when I need it."
- **Reflection:** "Asking for help is a sign of strength, not weakness."
- **Practical Exercise:** Identify a support system (e.g., friends, family, therapist). Reach out to them when you need support and reflect on the impact it has on your recovery.

May 31

- **Affirmation:** "I am committed to my self-care and

recovery journey."
- **Reflection:** "Commitment to self-care is a lifelong journey that supports your overall well-being."
- **Practical Exercise:** Reflect on the self-care practices you've implemented this month. Write about the progress you've made and set intentions for continuing your self-care journey.

May Conclusion

As we conclude this month focused on self-care and recovery, take a moment to reflect on the progress you have made in nurturing your mind, body, and spirit. Self-care is a continuous journey that requires dedication and commitment, but it is essential for your overall well-being. Over the past weeks, you have explored various self-care practices, developed a balanced self-care plan, and integrated journaling and meditation into your routine. Each of these steps has been a significant part of your healing and personal growth.

Throughout this month, you have learned to listen to your body's needs and respond with kindness, creating a self-care routine that supports your well-being. You have practiced self-compassion and forgiven yourself for any lapses, recognizing that growth is a journey. By acknowledging and expressing your emotions through journaling, you have gained deeper insights into your feelings and have set goals to track your progress.

You have balanced your self-care activities to nurture your whole self, addressing physical, emotional, mental, and spiritual needs. Whether through physical activities, emotional self-care practices, mental stimulation, or spiritual connections, each effort has contributed to your overall health and energy levels. You have also explored mindfulness and meditation, discovering techniques to stay present and connected, reduce stress, and find inner peace.

Remember to continue prioritizing your needs, seeking support when necessary, and being kind to yourself throughout this journey. Celebrate your progress, acknowledge your efforts, and invest in your self-care. You deserve to live a life that is fulfilling, balanced, and enriched by practices that support your recovery and overall happiness. Keep moving forward with confidence and self-compassion, knowing that each step you take brings you closer to a healthier and more vibrant life. Embrace the journey of self-care and recovery, and know that you have the tools and strength to continue on this path.

June: Getting Help When Needed

Seeking help when needed is a vital step in the journey toward healing and well-being. Recognizing when to seek help, understanding the types of support available, and learning how to access and utilize these resources effectively are all essential components of this process. Acknowledging that you need help and taking action to get it is a sign of strength and self-awareness.

Facing your pain is the first step toward healing. This involves acknowledging the pain, understanding its sources, and taking initial steps to confront and process it. By facing your pain head-on, you begin to understand its roots and start the healing process.

Understanding the importance of professional support is crucial. There are various types of mental health professionals, each offering different forms of assistance. Knowing how to advocate for your needs in these settings ensures you receive the support that best suits your situation. Professional support can offer valuable insights, coping strategies, and tools to manage your mental health effectively.

Coping strategies for depression include recognizing its symptoms, seeking support, and implementing self-care practices. Managing anxiety and stress involves learning techniques to reduce stress levels and create a balanced life. These strategies are essential for maintaining your mental and emotional health.

Building a support network is another critical aspect of managing your mental health. This network can include professional, personal, and community resources. A robust support network provides valuable assistance and comfort, helping you to navigate mental health challenges more effectively.

Remember, you do not have to navigate this journey alone. There are resources and support systems available to help you thrive. Each step you take toward seeking help and managing your mental health brings you closer to a healthier and more fulfilling life.

Week 1: Facing Your Pain

Introduction of Week's Theme

Facing your pain is the first and most crucial step toward healing and recovery. Embracing your pain involves acknowledging the hurt and suffering you have experienced without minimizing or dismissing it. Recognizing your pain fully is essential for healing, allowing yourself to experience and understand it. This acknowledgment is the first step toward releasing the hold that pain has on your life.

Understanding the sources of your pain is equally important. Pain can stem from various experiences, such as trauma, loss, or ongoing stress. Reflecting on these sources and how they have impacted your mental and emotional health provides clarity and insight into your healing journey.

Confronting and processing your pain requires courage and self-compassion. Approaching your pain with kindness and allowing yourself to feel and express your emotions without judgment breaks the cycle of suffering and opens the door to healing.

Self-compassion plays a vital role in facing your pain. Treat yourself with the same kindness and understanding that you would offer to a friend in distress. Recognize that your pain is valid and that you deserve care and support.

Strength is found in vulnerability. Embracing your vulnerabilities leads to greater resilience and personal growth. Seeing vulnerability not as a weakness but as a source of strength and authenticity is crucial for healing and building a more resilient self.

Seeking support is an important part of facing your pain. Whether from friends, family, or professional counselors, having a support system makes the process more manageable. Reaching out for support, sharing your experiences, and gaining comfort from those who understand and care about your well-being are essential steps.

Throughout this week, confront your painful experiences with kindness and courage, laying a strong foundation for your healing journey. By facing your pain directly, you take a powerful step toward a healthier and more fulfilling life.

June 1

- **Affirmation:** "I have the courage to face my pain and begin the healing process."
- **Reflection:** "Acknowledging your pain is a crucial step toward healing."
- **Practical Exercise:** Write about a painful experience that you have been avoiding. Reflect on how acknowledging this pain feels and any insights gained.

June 2

- **Affirmation:** "I will be kind to myself as I confront my pain."
- **Reflection:** "Self-compassion is essential when dealing with difficult emotions."
- **Practical Exercise:** Practice self-compassion by

writing a letter to yourself, offering kindness and understanding as you face your pain.

June 3

- **Affirmation:** "I can find strength in acknowledging my vulnerabilities."
- **Reflection:** "Embracing your vulnerabilities can lead to greater resilience and growth."
- **Practical Exercise:** Reflect on your vulnerabilities and how they have impacted your life. Write about how acknowledging them can help you grow stronger.

June 4

- **Affirmation:** "I will seek support as I face my pain."
- **Reflection:** "Seeking support can make the process of confronting your pain more manageable."
- **Practical Exercise:** Identify someone you trust (a friend, family member, or therapist) and share your experience of facing your pain with them.

June 5

- **Affirmation:** "I am not alone in my journey toward healing."
- **Reflection:** "Recognizing that you are not alone can provide comfort and strength."
- **Practical Exercise:** Join a support group or online community where you can share your experiences and connect with others who are facing similar challenges.

June 6

- **Affirmation:** "I will take small steps each day to face my pain."
- **Reflection:** "Healing is a gradual process that happens one step at a time."
- **Practical Exercise:** Identify one small step you can take each day to confront your pain. Reflect on your progress at the end of the week.

June 7

- **Affirmation:** "I trust the process of healing and give myself time to heal."

- **Reflection:** "Healing takes time and patience. Trust the journey."
- **Practical Exercise:** Create a timeline of your healing journey, noting key milestones and progress points. Reflect on the importance of patience in this process.

Week 2: Understanding the Importance of Getting Help

Introduction of Week's Theme

Seeking professional support is a crucial step in managing mental health challenges. Recognizing that you may need help from a trained professional is not a sign of weakness but a testament to your strength and commitment to your well-being. This week, we will explore the various forms of professional support available and provide guidance on how to access these valuable resources effectively.

Professional support can offer new perspectives and strategies that you might not have considered. Mental health professionals, such as therapists, counselors, and psychiatrists, are trained to understand complex emotional and psychological issues. They can provide you with tools and techniques to manage your mental health more effectively, helping you navigate through challenging times with greater resilience.

Being open to receiving help is an important part of the healing process. Sometimes, despite our best efforts, we need an external perspective to see things more clearly. This openness can lead to significant breakthroughs in understanding and managing your mental health. This week, we will focus on the importance of being receptive to professional help and how this can accelerate your journey toward healing.

Advocating for your needs in professional settings ensures you receive the support that is most beneficial to you. Clear communication with mental health professionals about your concerns, symptoms, and goals can lead to more tailored and effective care. We will discuss how to prepare for appointments, ask the right questions, and express your needs clearly.

Finding the right professional support can take time and persistence. It may involve meeting with different professionals to find the one that best suits your needs. This process requires patience, but the right match can make a significant difference in your mental health journey. We will offer practical advice on how to navigate this process and stay motivated.

Remember, you are worthy of receiving the help you need to thrive. Professional support is a valuable resource that can contribute significantly to your healing and personal growth. By seeking out and engaging with mental health professionals, you are taking a proactive step toward a healthier, more balanced life. This week, commit to exploring and utilizing the professional support available to you and embrace the positive changes it can bring to your mental health and overall well-being.

June 8

- **Affirmation:** "Seeking professional help is a sign of strength, not weakness."
- **Reflection:** "Professional support can offer new perspectives and effective strategies for healing."
- **Practical Exercise:** Research different types of mental health professionals (e.g., therapists, counselors, psychiatrists). Reflect on which type of support might be most beneficial for you.

June 9

- **Affirmation:** "I am open to receiving the help I need."
- **Reflection:** "Being open to help is an important part of the healing process."
- **Practical Exercise:** Make an appointment with a mental health professional or attend a consultation to explore your options for professional support.

June 10

- **Affirmation:** "I will advocate for my needs in professional settings."
- **Reflection:** "Effective communication with professionals ensures you receive the support you need."
- **Practical Exercise:** Prepare a list of questions and concerns to discuss with a mental health professional. Reflect on how advocating for your needs can improve your care.

June 11

- **Affirmation:** "I will be patient with myself as I seek professional support."
- **Reflection:** "Finding the right professional support can take time and persistence."
- **Practical Exercise:** Reflect on your journey to find professional support. Write about any challenges you have faced and how you can remain patient and persistent.

June 12

- **Affirmation:** "I deserve professional support to help me heal and grow."
- **Reflection:** "You are worthy of receiving the help you need to thrive."
- **Practical Exercise:** Write about why you deserve professional support and how it can contribute to your healing journey.

June 13

- **Affirmation:** "I will trust the expertise of the professionals I seek help from."
- **Reflection:** "Trusting in professional guidance is crucial for effective healing."
- **Practical Exercise:** Reflect on how trusting professionals can enhance your healing process. Write about a time when professional help made a significant impact on your well-being.

June 14

- **Affirmation:** "I am committed to finding the right professional support for my needs."
- **Reflection:** "Finding the right support is a journey worth committing to."
- **Practical Exercise:** Create a plan for seeking professional support, including potential professionals to contact and steps to take. Reflect on your commitment to this process.

Week 3: Coping with Sad Feelings and Depression

Introduction of Week's Theme

Sad feelings and depression are common mental health challenges that often stem from growing up in a toxic family environment. The negative messages about your value as a human being can leave deep scars on your sense of self-esteem and self-worth. This week, we will explore various strategies to cope with these feelings, helping you to recognize symptoms, seek appropriate support, and implement effective self-care practices.

Understanding and acknowledging the symptoms of depression is the first step toward managing it. Depression can manifest in many ways, including:

- Persistent sadness or a depressed mood
- Loss of interest or pleasure in activities once enjoyed
- Significant changes in appetite or weight (increase or decrease)
- Difficulty sleeping or oversleeping
- Fatigue or loss of energy
- Feelings of hopelessness or worthlessness
- Difficulty concentrating, making decisions, or remembering things
- Restlessness or irritability
- Physical symptoms such as aches, pains, or digestive

issues without a clear cause
- Thoughts of death or suicide

By becoming aware of these signs, you can take proactive steps to address them and seek the necessary help.

Seeking support is crucial when dealing with depression. It's important to reach out to trusted friends, family members, or professionals who can offer comfort, understanding, and guidance. Sharing your feelings and experiences with others can alleviate some of the emotional burdens and help you feel less isolated. This week, we will focus on identifying your support network and learning how to communicate your needs effectively.

Self-care practices play a vital role in managing depression. Incorporating activities that promote mental and emotional well-being into your daily routine can help alleviate symptoms and improve your overall mood. These practices can include regular exercise, healthy eating, mindfulness, and engaging in hobbies that bring you joy. We will explore various self-care strategies and how to integrate them into your life.

June 15
- **Affirmation:** "I will recognize the signs of depression and take steps to address it."
- **Reflection:** "Awareness of depression symptoms is the first step toward managing them."
- **Practical Exercise:** Reflect on any symptoms of depression you may be experiencing. Write about how recognizing these symptoms can help you seek appropriate support.

June 16
- **Affirmation:** "I am not defined by my depression; I can take steps to manage it."
- **Reflection:** "Depression is a condition, not an identity. You have the power to take action."
- **Practical Exercise:** Create a list of small, manageable

steps you can take to address your depression. Commit to taking one step today.

June 17

- **Affirmation:** "I will reach out for support when I feel overwhelmed."
- **Reflection:** "Reaching out for support is a crucial part of managing depression."
- **Practical Exercise:** Identify a trusted person you can reach out to when you feel overwhelmed. Make a plan to contact them when you need support.

June 18

- **Affirmation:** "I will incorporate self-care practices to help manage my depression."
- **Reflection:** "Self-care is an essential part of managing your mental health."
- **Practical Exercise:** Choose a self-care practice (e.g., exercise, journaling, meditation) and incorporate it into your daily routine. Reflect on its impact on your mood.

June 19

- **Affirmation:** "I will be gentle with myself as I navigate my journey with depression."
- **Reflection:** "Self-compassion is crucial when dealing with depression."
- **Practical Exercise:** Write a self-compassionate letter to yourself, acknowledging your struggles with depression and offering kindness and understanding.

June 20

- **Affirmation:** "I will monitor my progress and adjust my strategies as needed."
- **Reflection:** "Monitoring your progress helps you stay on track and make necessary adjustments."
- **Practical Exercise:** Keep a journal of your daily mood and activities. Reflect on what strategies are working and what might need to be adjusted.

June 21

- **Affirmation:** "I am capable of overcoming the challenges of depression."
- **Reflection:** "Believing in your ability to overcome challenges is empowering."
- **Practical Exercise:** Write about a time when you overcame a significant challenge. Reflect on how that experience can inspire you to manage your depression.

Week 4: Managing Anxiety and Stress

Introduction of Week's Theme

Anxiety and stress are prevalent issues that many people face in their daily lives. They can stem from various sources, such as work, relationships, health concerns, and personal challenges. Understanding how to manage these feelings is crucial for maintaining mental and emotional well-being. This week, we will explore effective strategies for coping with anxiety and stress, aiming to help you cultivate a calmer and more balanced life.

Recognizing the signs of anxiety and stress is the first step toward managing them. Symptoms can include persistent worry, irritability, difficulty concentrating, muscle tension, and sleep disturbances. By becoming aware of these signs, you can take proactive steps to address them before they escalate. This awareness will empower you to respond to stressors in a healthier and more controlled manner.

One of the most effective ways to manage anxiety and stress is through relaxation techniques. Practices such as deep breathing, progressive muscle relaxation, and guided imagery can significantly reduce stress levels. These techniques help calm the mind and body, providing immediate relief from tension and anxiety. This week, we will explore various relaxation methods and encourage you to integrate them into your daily routine.

Another important strategy is to create a structured plan to manage stress and anxiety. Having a clear plan can make you feel more in control and reduce the overwhelming nature of stressors. This plan might include identifying triggers, developing coping strategies, and setting realistic goals. By taking a systematic approach, you can tackle anxiety and stress in a more organized and effective way.

Support systems play a crucial role in managing anxiety and stress. Reaching out to friends, family members, or support groups can provide much-needed comfort and perspective. Sharing your feelings and experiences with others can alleviate the burden of anxiety and make you feel less isolated. This week, we will focus on the importance of building and utilizing a strong support network.

Incorporating mindfulness practices into your life can also help manage anxiety and stress. Mindfulness involves staying present in the moment and observing your thoughts and feelings without judgment. Techniques such as mindful breathing and body scanning can help ground you and reduce anxiety. By practicing mindfulness regularly, you can develop a greater sense of peace and resilience.

Lastly, maintaining physical health through regular exercise and good sleep hygiene is essential for managing stress and anxiety. Physical activity releases endorphins, which can improve mood and reduce stress levels. Additionally, establishing a healthy sleep routine can significantly impact your mental health. This week, we will discuss the importance of exercise and sleep in managing anxiety and provide practical tips for incorporating them into your daily life.

June 22
- **Affirmation:** "I will recognize the signs of anxiety and take steps to manage it."
- **Reflection:** "Awareness of anxiety symptoms is the first step toward managing them."

- **Practical Exercise:** Reflect on any symptoms of anxiety you may be experiencing. Write about how recognizing these symptoms can help you seek appropriate support.

June 23

- **Affirmation:** "I can use relaxation techniques to reduce my stress levels."
- **Reflection:** "Relaxation techniques can help you manage stress and anxiety effectively."
- **Practical Exercise:** Practice a relaxation technique, such as deep breathing, progressive muscle relaxation, or guided imagery. Reflect on its impact on your stress levels.

June 24

- **Affirmation:** "I will create a plan to manage my stress and anxiety."
- **Reflection:** "Having a plan in place can help you feel more in control of your anxiety and stress."
- **Practical Exercise:** Create a stress management plan that includes triggers, coping strategies, and support resources. Reflect on how having a plan can help you manage your anxiety and stress.

June 25

- **Affirmation:** "I will seek support from others to help manage my anxiety and stress."
- **Reflection:** "Support from others can provide comfort and perspective."
- **Practical Exercise:** Reach out to a friend, family member, or support group to share your experiences with anxiety and stress. Reflect on the support you receive and how it helps you cope.

June 26

- **Affirmation:** "I will practice mindfulness to stay present and reduce anxiety."
- **Reflection:** "Mindfulness helps you stay grounded and focused on the present moment."
- **Practical Exercise:** Practice a mindfulness exercise,

such as mindful breathing or body scan. Reflect on how staying present affects your anxiety levels.

June 27

- **Affirmation:** "I will incorporate regular physical activity to manage my anxiety and stress."
- **Reflection:** "Physical activity can help reduce anxiety and stress levels."
- **Practical Exercise:** Choose a physical activity you enjoy and incorporate it into your routine. Reflect on its impact on your mood and stress levels.

June 28

- **Affirmation:** "I will establish a healthy sleep routine to support my mental health."
- **Reflection:** "Good sleep hygiene is essential for managing anxiety and stress."
- **Practical Exercise:** Create a sleep routine that promotes good sleep hygiene, such as maintaining a consistent bedtime and creating a calming pre-sleep ritual. Reflect on how improving your sleep habits affects your anxiety and stress levels.

June 29

- **Affirmation:** "I will use my support network to help manage my anxiety and stress."
- **Reflection:** "Your support network can provide valuable assistance and comfort during stressful times."
- **Practical Exercise:** List the people and resources in your support network. Reach out to one person or resource today and share how they can support you in managing your anxiety and stress.

June 30

- **Affirmation:** "I am grateful for the support I receive in managing my anxiety and stress."
- **Reflection:** "Gratitude for your support system can help reduce anxiety and promote a positive mindset."
- **Practical Exercise:** Write a gratitude list focusing on the support you have received and the progress you

have made in managing your anxiety and stress this month. Reflect on how gratitude enhances your well-being and helps alleviate anxiety.

June Conclusion

As we conclude this month focused on getting help when needed, take a moment to reflect on the significant progress you have made. Recognizing the importance of support and taking concrete steps to seek it is a powerful act of self-care and resilience. By acknowledging when you need help and reaching out for support, you have demonstrated immense courage and a commitment to your well-being.

This month, you have faced your pain head-on, learning to acknowledge and confront it rather than avoid it. This is a crucial first step in the healing process, allowing you to begin addressing the underlying issues that have caused you distress. Your willingness to face your vulnerabilities has paved the way for greater resilience and personal growth.

Understanding the importance of professional support has been another key focus. You have explored the various types of mental health professionals and learned how to access the help you need. By seeking professional guidance, you have taken an essential step toward gaining new perspectives and effective strategies for managing your mental health challenges.

You have also developed strategies to cope with depression, recognizing its symptoms and taking actionable steps to manage it. Incorporating self-care practices and reaching out for support when feeling overwhelmed are significant strides in prioritizing your mental health. Your efforts in managing depression highlight your determination to take control of your well-being.

In managing anxiety and stress, you have practiced techniques such as mindfulness, relaxation exercises, and creating stress management plans. These practices have helped you reduce anxiety and maintain a sense of calm and balance in your life. By identifying and utilizing your support network, you have recognized the invaluable assistance and comfort that others can provide during stressful times.

Reflect on the skills you have acquired this month:

- **Facing Pain:** You have learned to acknowledge your pain and begin the healing process.
- **Professional Support:** You have explored the value of professional help and how to access it.
- **Coping with Depression:** You have developed strategies to manage depression and prioritize self-care.
- **Managing Anxiety and Stress:** You have practiced techniques to reduce anxiety and stress, enhancing your mental health.
- **Utilizing Support Systems:** You have identified and strengthened your support network, recognizing its importance in your healing journey.

Celebrate your progress, acknowledge your strength, and continue to prioritize your well-being. Each step you take brings you closer to a healthier and more fulfilling life. Keep moving forward with confidence and self-compassion, knowing that you are on a path to recovery and growth. Thank you for dedicating this month to your well-being. Your commitment to healing and seeking support is truly inspiring. Here's to your continued growth and the bright future that lies ahead.

July: Stop Toxic Thinking

Toxic thinking patterns can significantly impact your mental health and overall well-being, often leading to feelings of low self-esteem, chronic stress, and a pervasive sense of negativity. These detrimental thoughts can become deeply ingrained, influencing how you perceive yourself and interact with the world. This month, we will focus on identifying and challenging these negative thought patterns and replacing them with healthier and more constructive ways of thinking. By addressing toxic thoughts head-on, you can pave the way for a more balanced, optimistic, and fulfilling life.

Recognizing toxic thinking is the first crucial step toward transformation. Many of these patterns, such as catastrophizing, overgeneralizing, and self-criticism, can go unnoticed because they have become habitual. This month, we will explore these common toxic thought patterns, helping you understand their origins and how they manifest in your daily life. Awareness is key, as it allows you to catch these thoughts before they take root and cause further emotional harm.

Once you have identified these harmful thought patterns, the next step is to challenge and reframe them. Cognitive restructuring, a technique used in cognitive-behavioral therapy (CBT), will be a central focus. This method involves questioning the validity of negative thoughts and replacing them with more realistic and positive alternatives. By learning to dispute and change these thoughts, you can break the cycle of negativity and foster a more supportive internal dialogue.

Mindfulness will also play a pivotal role in this month's journey. Mindfulness practices help you become more aware of your thoughts without judgment, allowing you to observe them from a distance rather than getting caught up in them. This non-reactive awareness can help you identify toxic thoughts as they arise and choose how to respond to them rather than being driven by automatic negative reactions. Mindfulness can also anchor you in the present moment, reducing the tendency to ruminate on past mistakes or worry excessively about the future.

Positive affirmations will be another powerful tool in our arsenal against toxic thinking. Affirmations are positive statements that you repeat to yourself to challenge and overcome self-sabotaging and negative thoughts. They can help rewire your brain, fostering a more positive self-image and outlook on life. This month, you will learn how to create and effectively use affirmations to counteract negativity and build a more resilient mindset.

In addition to these techniques, we will explore practical strategies for maintaining a positive mental environment. This includes setting boundaries to protect yourself from external negativity, engaging in activities that uplift and inspire you, and surrounding yourself with supportive, positive influences. By integrating these practices into your daily routine, you can create a mental environment that supports your well-being and personal growth.

Week 1: Identifying Toxic Thoughts

Introduction of Week's Theme

The journey to overcoming toxic thinking begins with identifying the negative thought patterns that are detrimental to your mental well-being. These toxic thoughts often operate beneath the surface of our conscious mind, subtly influencing our emotions, behaviors, and overall outlook on life. This week, our focus will be on bringing these harmful thought patterns to light, understanding their origins, and recognizing their profound impact on our mental health.

Toxic thoughts can manifest in various forms, such as self-criticism, catastrophic thinking, and persistent doubt. These thoughts are often deeply ingrained, shaped by past experiences, and reinforced over time. By identifying and acknowledging these patterns, you can start to break their hold on your mind and create space for healthier, more constructive thoughts. This awareness is a crucial first step in your journey toward mental clarity and emotional freedom.

Throughout this week, we will explore practical exercises to help you become more aware of your thoughts. Keeping a thought journal can be a powerful tool in this process. By writing down your recurring negative thoughts, you can start to see patterns and understand how these thoughts are impacting your mood and behavior. Reflecting on these entries will provide valuable insights into the specific thoughts that need to be addressed and challenged.

Understanding the sources of your toxic thoughts is another important aspect of this week's theme. These thoughts often stem from past experiences, societal pressures, or internalized beliefs that no longer serve you. By examining the origins of your negative thinking, you can begin to dismantle the false narratives that have been holding you back. This process requires honesty and self-compassion, as it involves confronting parts of yourself that may be painful or uncomfortable.

We will also explore the concept of cognitive distortions, which are irrational thought patterns that can perpetuate toxic thinking. Common cognitive distortions include black-and-white thinking, overgeneralization, and filtering out the positive. Learning to identify these distortions in your thinking will empower you to challenge and reframe them, ultimately leading to a more balanced and realistic perspective.

As you progress through this week, remember that changing your thought patterns is a gradual process. Be patient with yourself and acknowledge the small victories along the way. Each step you take in recognizing and addressing your toxic thoughts brings you closer to a healthier, more positive mindset. Engage fully with the exercises and reflections provided, and trust that this foundational work is setting the stage for lasting change.

By the end of this week, you will have developed a greater awareness of your toxic thoughts and their impact on your life. This awareness is the first crucial step in transforming your mental landscape. Embrace this journey with an open heart and mind, knowing that you are taking meaningful steps toward greater mental clarity and emotional well-being.

You are not your thoughts or emotions; you are the consciousness experiencing them. Observe your thoughts and feelings, as if from a distance, as they come and go, like waves on the seashore. Avoid becoming too attached to them, as they may seem crucial now but will eventually pass. You are the being that remains in the stillness.

July 1
- **Affirmation:** "I am aware of my thoughts and can recognize toxic patterns."
- **Reflection:** "Awareness is the first step to change."
- **Practical Exercise:** Write down recurring negative thoughts you have throughout the day. Reflect on how these thoughts affect your emotions and behavior.

July 2
- **Affirmation:** "I can distinguish between helpful and harmful thoughts."

- **Reflection:** "Not all thoughts serve your well-being. Learning to distinguish them is crucial."
- **Practical Exercise:** Review your list of recurring negative thoughts from yesterday. Identify which ones are harmful and which ones, if any, are helpful.

July 3

- **Affirmation:** "I will challenge the validity of my toxic thoughts."
- **Reflection:** "Many negative thoughts are based on distorted thinking rather than reality."
- **Practical Exercise:** Choose one negative thought and challenge its validity. Ask yourself questions like, "Is this thought based on facts?" and "What evidence do I have to support or refute it?"

July 4

- **Affirmation:** "I have the power to change my thought patterns."
- **Reflection:** "You are in control of your thoughts and can change them for the better."
- **Practical Exercise:** Write about a situation where you successfully changed a negative thought into a positive one. Reflect on how it affected your emotions and behavior.

July 5

- **Affirmation:** "I will not let negative thoughts dictate my actions."
- **Reflection:** "You can choose to act differently, regardless of your negative thoughts."
- **Practical Exercise:** Identify a negative thought that often dictates your actions. Plan a different, positive action you can take the next time this thought arises.

July 6

- **Affirmation:** "I am in control of my thoughts and can redirect them."
- **Reflection:** "Redirecting your thoughts can help you maintain a positive mindset."
- **Practical Exercise:** Practice redirecting a negative

thought by focusing on a positive or neutral thought instead. Reflect on how this practice changes your emotional state.

July 7

- **Affirmation:** "I will replace negative thoughts with positive affirmations."
- **Reflection:** "Positive affirmations can help reframe your mindset."
- **Practical Exercise:** Create a list of positive affirmations to counteract your common negative thoughts. Repeat these affirmations daily and reflect on their impact.

Week 2: Avoiding Stress-Inducing Thoughts

Introduction of Week's Theme

Stress-inducing thoughts can significantly impact your mental health, leading to heightened anxiety and feelings of being overwhelmed. This week, our focus is on understanding how these thoughts manifest, identifying their triggers, and implementing strategies to manage and avoid them. By learning to control stress-inducing thoughts, you can cultivate a calmer, more balanced mindset that supports your overall well-being.

Recognize the common sources of stress-inducing thoughts. These can include worries about the future, ruminations on past events, and negative self-talk. Each of these sources can trigger a cascade of stress responses in your body, leading to physical symptoms such as increased heart rate and muscle tension, as well as emotional symptoms like anxiety and irritability. Understanding these triggers is the first step toward managing them effectively.

Become more aware of your stress triggers by keeping a journal of situations that cause you stress and the thoughts associated with them. This practice of self-reflection can help you pinpoint specific situations or thoughts that consistently induce stress, enabling you to address them more proactively.

One powerful method to combat stress-inducing thoughts is the practice of mindfulness. Mindfulness involves staying present in the moment and observing your thoughts without judgment. By focusing on the present, you can reduce the impact of stress-inducing thoughts that often stem from worries about the past or future. Explore different mindfulness exercises, such as mindful breathing and body scans, to help you develop this valuable skill.

Positive affirmations and thought redirection are also important. Positive affirmations can help counteract negative thought patterns and reinforce a calmer mindset. Redirecting your thoughts toward positive or neutral topics when you notice stress-inducing thoughts can be highly effective. These techniques can help you break the cycle of stress and create a more positive mental environment.

Self-care practices play a crucial role in managing stress. Activities such as regular exercise, proper sleep, and engaging in hobbies you enjoy can significantly reduce your stress levels. Identify self-care activities that work best for you and discuss how to incorporate them into your daily routine. These practices not only help manage stress in the moment but also build resilience against future stress.

July 8

- **Affirmation:** "I will recognize thoughts that trigger my stress."
- **Reflection:** "Identifying stress triggers helps you manage them effectively."
- **Practical Exercise:** Keep a journal of situations that cause you stress and the thoughts associated with them. Reflect on patterns you notice.

July 9

- **Affirmation:** "I can redirect my focus away from stress-inducing thoughts."

- **Reflection:** "Redirecting your focus can help reduce stress and anxiety."
- **Practical Exercise:** Practice redirecting your focus when a stress-inducing thought arises. Choose a positive or neutral topic to think about instead.

July 10

- **Affirmation:** "I will practice deep breathing to calm my mind."
- **Reflection:** "Deep breathing helps reduce the physical symptoms of stress."
- **Practical Exercise:** Practice deep breathing exercises for five minutes when you notice stress-inducing thoughts. Reflect on the impact on your stress levels.

July 11

- **Affirmation:** "I can create a mental environment that fosters calmness."
- **Reflection:** "A calm mental environment helps you handle stress more effectively."
- **Practical Exercise:** Create a calming mental environment by visualizing a peaceful place or repeating a calming mantra. Practice this visualization or mantra daily.

July 12

- **Affirmation:** "I will use positive affirmations to counteract stress-inducing thoughts."
- **Reflection:** "Positive affirmations can help shift your mindset from stress to calm."
- **Practical Exercise:** Write down three positive affirmations to counteract your most common stress-inducing thoughts. Repeat these affirmations daily.

July 13

- **Affirmation:** "I will practice mindfulness to stay present and reduce stress."
- **Reflection:** "Mindfulness helps you stay grounded and focused on the present moment."
- **Practical Exercise:** Practice a mindfulness exercise, such as mindful breathing or body scan. Reflect on how

staying present affects your stress levels.

July 14
- **Affirmation**: "I will prioritize self-care to manage stress effectively."
- **Reflection**: "Self-care is essential for maintaining a healthy stress response."
- **Practical Exercise**: Identify a self-care activity that helps you relax and reduce stress. Schedule time for this activity daily and reflect on its impact.

Week 3: Cognitive Errors and Negative Core Beliefs

Introduction of Week's Theme

Cognitive errors and negative core beliefs are often at the root of toxic thinking patterns, significantly impacting how we perceive ourselves and the world around us. These distorted thought patterns can lead to a cycle of negativity, undermining our self-esteem and overall well-being. This week, our focus will be on identifying these cognitive distortions and the negative core beliefs that drive them. By understanding and challenging these errors, we can replace them with healthier, more constructive alternatives.

Cognitive errors, also known as cognitive distortions, are irrational thought patterns that can lead to false conclusions and perpetuate negative thinking. Recognizing these errors is the first step toward correcting them and fostering a healthier mindset. Here are some common cognitive errors:

- Black-and-white thinking: Viewing situations in extreme, either-or terms.
- Overgeneralization: Drawing broad conclusions from a single event.
- Catastrophizing: Expecting the worst possible outcome in any situation.
- Personalization: Blaming yourself for events outside

your control.
- Mind reading: Assuming you know what others are thinking without evidence.
- Should statements: Rigid rules about how you and others must behave.
- Discounting the positive: Ignoring or dismissing positive experiences.

Negative core beliefs are deeply ingrained perceptions about ourselves, others, and the world that are often formed in childhood and reinforced over time. These beliefs influence our thoughts, feelings, and behaviors, often leading to self-sabotage and limiting our potential for growth and happiness. Here are some examples of negative core beliefs:

- "I am not good enough."
- "I will always fail."
- "The world is a dangerous place."
- "People cannot be trusted."
- "I am unlovable."
- "I don't deserve happiness."
- "I don't deserve success."
- "I don't deserve a loving partner."
- "I am powerless."

Exercises can help identify and understand cognitive errors and negative core beliefs. By bringing these patterns to light, you can begin to see how they influence your daily thoughts and actions. This awareness is crucial for initiating change and breaking free from the cycle of negativity that these distortions perpetuate.

Techniques to challenge and reframe cognitive errors and negative core beliefs include questioning the validity of these thoughts and beliefs, gathering evidence for and against them, and considering more balanced and realistic alternatives. Here are some examples of positive core beliefs to replace the negative ones:

- "I am worthy of love and respect."

- "I am capable and competent."
- "The world is full of opportunities."
- "People can be kind and supportive."
- "I deserve happiness and fulfillment."
- "I have the power to change my life."
- "I am resilient and strong."

Self-compassion plays a vital role in this process. Challenging deeply held beliefs and thought patterns can be a difficult and emotional journey. Self-compassion allows you to approach this work with kindness and understanding rather than self-criticism and judgment. It is essential to treat yourself with the same care and respect you would offer a close friend going through a similar process.

By understanding your cognitive errors and negative core beliefs and acquiring tools and strategies to challenge and reframe these thoughts, you can pave the way for a healthier, more positive mindset. Remember, changing thought patterns takes time and persistence, but each step you take brings you closer to mental clarity and emotional resilience. Let's embark on this transformative journey together, with patience and self-compassion, as we work toward eliminating toxic thinking and embracing a healthier perspective.

July 15

- **Affirmation:** "I am aware of cognitive errors that distort my thinking."
- **Reflection:** "Recognizing cognitive errors is the first step to correcting them."
- **Practical Exercise:** Learn about common cognitive errors (e.g., black-and-white thinking, overgeneralization). Identify which ones you often make and write about examples from your life.

July 16

- **Affirmation:** "I will challenge and reframe my cognitive errors."
- **Reflection:** "Challenging cognitive errors helps you

develop healthier thought patterns."
- **Practical Exercise:** Choose one cognitive error you identified yesterday. Challenge and reframe it using evidence and logical reasoning.

July 17

- **Affirmation:** "I will identify and question my negative core beliefs."
- **Reflection:** "Negative core beliefs often drive toxic thinking. Questioning them is crucial."
- **Practical Exercise:** Write down a negative core belief you hold about yourself. Question its validity by asking, "What evidence do I have for this belief?" and "Is there an alternative, more positive belief I could adopt?"

July 18

- **Affirmation:** "I can replace negative core beliefs with positive ones."
- **Reflection:** "Replacing negative beliefs with positive ones can transform your mindset."
- **Practical Exercise:** Rewrite the negative core belief you identified yesterday into a positive one. Repeat this new belief to yourself daily and reflect on any changes in your mindset.

July 19

- **Affirmation:** "I will practice self-compassion to counteract negative beliefs."
- **Reflection:** "Self-compassion helps you challenge and change negative core beliefs."
- **Practical Exercise:** Write a self-compassionate letter to yourself, addressing the negative core belief you are working to change. Reflect on how this exercise makes you feel.

July 20

- **Affirmation:** "I will replace negative self-talk with positive affirmations."
- **Reflection:** "Positive affirmations can counteract negative self-talk and boost self-esteem."

- **Practical Exercise:** Identify negative self-talk patterns. Write positive affirmations to replace them and practice these affirmations daily.

July 21

- **Affirmation:** "I am committed to changing my thought patterns for the better."
- **Reflection:** "Commitment to positive change is essential for long-term transformation."
- **Practical Exercise:** Reflect on your commitment to changing negative thought patterns. Write about the progress you have made and set goals for continued improvement.

Week 4: Mindfulness to Eliminate Toxic Thinking

Introduction of Week's Theme

Mindfulness is a powerful tool for recognizing and managing toxic thoughts, helping you stay present, reduce the impact of negative thinking, and cultivate a more positive mindset. It involves paying attention to the present moment without judgment, allowing you to observe your thoughts and feelings as they arise. This heightened awareness helps you recognize negative thoughts before they spiral out of control.

One of the key benefits of mindfulness is its ability to reduce stress and anxiety. By focusing on the here and now, you are less likely to get caught up in worries about the past or future, which can fuel toxic thinking. This shift in focus can significantly improve your mental well-being and help you develop a more balanced perspective.

Incorporating mindfulness into your daily routine can help you build resilience against negative thinking. Practices such as mindful breathing, meditation, and body scans ground you in the present moment and create a sense of inner peace. These practices not only reduce the immediate impact of toxic thoughts but also strengthen your overall mental health, making you more resistant to stress and negativity in the long term.

Observing your thoughts without judgment is essential. Recognize them as temporary mental events rather than absolute truths. This detachment reduces their emotional impact and prevents them from controlling your mood and behavior. Techniques such as mindful breathing and body scans anchor you in the now, promoting a sense of calm and clarity.

Cultivating a compassionate mindset involves responding to your thoughts with kindness rather than criticism. This shift in perspective diminishes the power of toxic thoughts and fosters a healthier mental landscape. Mindfulness is a skill that develops over time, so be patient and persistent. Progress may be gradual, but each practice session strengthens your ability to manage negative thinking.

By consistently applying these mindfulness techniques, you can transform your relationship with your thoughts, reducing their hold on you and enhancing your overall mental well-being. Embrace this opportunity to cultivate a positive mindset and take a significant step toward a healthier, more fulfilling life.

July 22

- **Affirmation:** "I will practice mindfulness to become aware of my thoughts."
- **Reflection:** "Mindfulness helps you observe your thoughts without judgment."
- **Practical Exercise:** Practice a mindfulness meditation focused on observing your thoughts. Notice any toxic thoughts that arise and let them pass without judgment.

July 23

- **Affirmation:** "I can stay present and focused in the moment."

- **Reflection:** "Staying present helps reduce the impact of toxic thoughts."
- **Practical Exercise:** Practice mindful breathing, focusing on your breath as it moves in and out. When your mind wanders, gently bring it back to your breath.

July 24

- **Affirmation:** "I will use mindfulness to reduce the power of negative thoughts."
- **Reflection:** "Mindfulness can diminish the hold of negative thoughts on your mind."
- **Practical Exercise:** Throughout the day, practice bringing your attention back to the present moment whenever you notice a negative thought. Reflect on how this practice affects your mindset.

July 25

- **Affirmation:** "I will cultivate a non-judgmental attitude toward my thoughts."
- **Reflection:** "Non-judgmental awareness helps you accept your thoughts without being controlled by them."
- **Practical Exercise:** Practice observing your thoughts without labeling them as good or bad. Reflect on how this non-judgmental attitude impacts your mental state.

July 26

- **Affirmation:** "I will incorporate mindfulness into my daily routine."
- **Reflection:** "Regular mindfulness practice supports mental clarity and emotional balance."
- **Practical Exercise:** Set aside time each day for a mindfulness practice, such as mindful eating, walking, or meditation. Reflect on the changes you notice in your thoughts and emotions.

July 27

- **Affirmation:** "I am present, aware, and in control of my thoughts."

- **Reflection:** "Mindfulness empowers you to take control of your mental state."
- **Practical Exercise:** Practice a body scan meditation to connect with your body and stay present. Reflect on how this practice helps you feel more grounded and in control.

July 28

- **Affirmation:** "I will practice gratitude to shift my focus to the positive."
- **Reflection:** "Gratitude helps redirect your focus from negative to positive thoughts."
- **Practical Exercise:** Write a daily gratitude list, noting at least three things you are grateful for each day. Reflect on how this practice affects your mindset.

July 29

- **Affirmation:** "I will use positive affirmations to reshape my thinking."
- **Reflection:** "Positive affirmations can help rewire your brain for a more positive outlook."
- **Practical Exercise:** Write down five positive affirmations that resonate with you. Repeat them daily and reflect on any changes in your mindset.

July 30

- **Affirmation:** "I can visualize my success and happiness."
- **Reflection:** "Visualization helps you create a positive mental image of your goals."
- **Practical Exercise:** Spend five minutes each day visualizing yourself achieving your goals and experiencing happiness. Reflect on how this practice influences your motivation and mood.

July 31

- **Affirmation:** "I am committed to maintaining a positive and healthy mindset."
- **Reflection:** "Commitment to positive thinking supports long-term mental well-being."
- **Practical Exercise:** Reflect on the progress you have

made this month in stopping toxic thinking. Write about the positive changes you have experienced and set intentions for continuing this practice.

July Conclusion

As we conclude this transformative month focused on stopping toxic thinking, take a moment to reflect deeply on the remarkable progress you have made in reshaping your thought patterns. The journey of identifying, challenging, and replacing toxic thoughts with positive and empowering ones is ongoing and requires continuous dedication and self-awareness. Recognize the strength and resilience you have demonstrated by committing to this vital aspect of mental well-being.

Over the past weeks, you have developed a keen awareness of your thoughts, learning to recognize the negative patterns that have been holding you back. Identifying these toxic thoughts is the first and most crucial step toward change. By becoming more aware of these patterns, you have taken control of your mental narrative, paving the way for healthier and more constructive thinking.

Challenging cognitive errors and negative core beliefs has been another significant achievement this month. You have learned to question the validity of distorted thinking and replace it with more rational and positive perspectives. This critical skill helps in dismantling deeply ingrained negative beliefs, allowing you to build a foundation of healthier, more empowering thoughts. This process is transformative, fostering a more optimistic outlook on life.

Mindfulness has played a pivotal role in your journey, enabling you to stay present and manage negative thinking effectively. By incorporating mindfulness practices into your daily routine, you have cultivated a non-judgmental awareness of your thoughts. This practice has helped you observe and let go of toxic thoughts without letting them control your emotions and actions. The mindfulness techniques you have learned will continue to support your mental well-being long after this month.

The use of positive affirmations and visualization has further strengthened your ability to cultivate a positive mindset. By regularly engaging in these practices, you have reinforced your self-worth and visualized your success and happiness. Positive affirmations and visualization are powerful tools that help rewire your brain for positivity, boosting your confidence and motivation.

Celebrate the significant progress you have made this month. Acknowledge the strength, resilience, and commitment you have shown in prioritizing your mental well-being. Continue to move forward with confidence and self-compassion, knowing that each step you take brings you closer to a more positive and empowered mindset. Your dedication to stopping toxic thinking and fostering a positive mental outlook is truly inspiring.

August: Rebuilding Self-Esteem

Rebuilding self-esteem is a critical aspect of healing from toxic relationships and environments. Self-esteem forms the foundation of how we perceive ourselves and our capabilities, influencing our decisions, behaviors, and overall quality of life. This month, we will explore understanding what self-esteem truly means, its importance in our lives, and how past experiences, particularly those involving toxic relationships, can erode this essential aspect of our identity. By recognizing these impacts, we can begin the transformative process of reclaiming and rebuilding our self-worth.

Past experiences, especially those involving toxic family dynamics, can significantly damage self-esteem. Constant criticism, unrealistic expectations, neglect, and emotional manipulation can leave lasting scars, creating a negative self-image and fostering self-doubt. This month, we will focus on identifying these detrimental influences and understanding how they have shaped your self-perception. Acknowledging the root causes of low self-esteem is the first step toward healing and rebuilding a stronger sense of self.

Rebuilding self-esteem involves not only addressing past wounds but also actively cultivating self-compassion and self-acceptance. We will explore techniques to nurture a positive self-image, including daily affirmations, self-care practices, and cognitive restructuring. These strategies will help you challenge negative self-beliefs and replace them with empowering positive thoughts. By integrating these practices into your daily routine, you will gradually strengthen your self-esteem and foster a healthier, more resilient mindset.

Developing self-esteem is an ongoing journey that requires patience, commitment, and self-awareness. This month, we will introduce practical exercises to help you track your progress, celebrate your achievements, and stay motivated. By setting realistic goals and acknowledging your growth, you can build a solid foundation of self-worth that supports your overall well-being. Remember, rebuilding self-esteem is not about perfection but about progress and self-improvement.

Support from others plays a crucial role in rebuilding self-esteem. Engaging with supportive friends, family, or support groups can provide encouragement, validation, and a sense of belonging. This month, we will discuss how to seek and accept support from others and how to create a positive and nurturing social environment. By surrounding yourself with people who uplift and inspire you, you can reinforce your efforts to build a healthier self-esteem.

Finally, we will explore the broader impacts of improved self-esteem on various aspects of your life. Enhanced self-esteem can lead to better relationships, increased resilience, and a more optimistic outlook on life. As you rebuild your self-esteem, you will likely notice positive changes in your personal and professional life, as well as in your ability to cope with challenges and pursue your goals. This month, commit to the journey of self-discovery and self-empowerment, embracing the opportunity to reclaim your self-worth and unlock your true potential.

Week 1: Recognizing Your Self-Worth

Understanding and recognizing your inherent worth is

the cornerstone of rebuilding self-esteem and fostering a healthy, positive self-image. Recognizing your worth is not about arrogance or superiority; it is about understanding and appreciating your unique qualities, strengths, and contributions.

Self-worth influences how you view yourself, interact with others, and navigate the world. When you understand your worth, you are less likely to seek validation from external sources and more likely to find confidence and contentment within yourself.

Internal and external factors shape your perception of self-worth. Many of us have internalized negative messages from our past, whether from family, society, or personal experiences. These messages can distort our self-perception and lead us to undervalue ourselves. Bringing these influences to light allows you to challenge and change them.

Practical exercises and techniques help you recognize and affirm your worth. These include journaling exercises to reflect on your strengths and achievements, affirmations to reinforce positive self-perceptions, and mindfulness practices to cultivate self-awareness. Consistently engaging in these activities can shift your mindset and build a stronger sense of self-worth.

Self-compassion plays a crucial role in recognizing your worth. Often, we are our own harshest critics, focusing on our perceived flaws and failures. Practicing self-compassion involves treating yourself with the same kindness and understanding you would offer a friend. This shift in perspective helps you see yourself in a more balanced and accepting light, recognizing that you are worthy of love and respect just as you are.

Daily affirmations and reflections support this journey. Take small, meaningful steps toward recognizing and embracing your worth. Aim to have a clearer understanding of your intrinsic value and a toolkit of strategies to maintain and nurture your self-worth moving forward.

Recognizing your worth is a continuous process that requires patience and commitment. It is a journey of self-discovery and growth that will empower you to live a more fulfilling and authentic life. Embrace the incredible journey of understanding and celebrating your inherent worth.

August 1

- **Affirmation:** "I am worthy of love and respect."
- **Reflection:** "Your worth is inherent and not dependent on external validation."
- **Practical Exercise:** Write down three things you value about yourself. Reflect on how these qualities contribute to your worth.

August 2

- **Affirmation:** "I will treat myself with kindness and compassion."
- **Reflection:** "Kindness and compassion toward yourself are vital for recognizing your worth."
- **Practical Exercise:** Practice self-compassion by writing a letter to yourself, acknowledging your worth and offering support and understanding.

August 3

- **Affirmation:** "I am enough just as I am."
- **Reflection:** "You are complete and whole just as you are. Embrace your uniqueness."
- **Practical Exercise:** Reflect on the statement "I am enough." Write about what this means to you and how you can remind yourself of this truth daily.

August 4

- **Affirmation:** "I deserve to prioritize my needs and well-being."
- **Reflection:** "Prioritizing your needs is a form of self-respect."

- **Practical Exercise:** Identify a need you have been neglecting. Take a step today to address and prioritize this need.

August 5
- **Affirmation:** "I will celebrate my achievements, no matter how small."
- **Reflection:** "Every achievement is a testament to your abilities and worth."
- **Practical Exercise:** Write down recent achievements, big or small. Reflect on how these accomplishments contribute to your sense of self-worth.

August 6
- **Affirmation:** "I believe in my abilities and strengths."
- **Reflection:** "Believing in yourself is crucial for building self-esteem."
- **Practical Exercise:** Write down affirmations that resonate with you and place them where you can see them daily. Repeat them each morning and night.

August 7
- **Affirmation:** "I am proud of who I am becoming."
- **Reflection:** "Acknowledge your growth and the person you are becoming."
- **Practical Exercise:** Reflect on your personal growth over the past year. Write about the positive changes you have made and how they contribute to your self-esteem.

Week 2: Positive Affirmations for Self-Esteem

Positive affirmations are powerful tools for reinforcing self-esteem and building a positive self-image. Affirmations are simple yet profound statements that can reshape your thoughts and beliefs, helping you cultivate a more empowering and nurturing inner dialogue.

Understanding the science behind affirmations is crucial. Affirmations work by reprogramming your subconscious mind, replacing negative self-talk with positive, self-affirming messages. When practiced consistently, these statements can lead to significant improvements in your self-esteem and overall mental health.

Creating effective affirmations requires intention and mindfulness. Craft personalized affirmations that resonate with your unique experiences and aspirations. These affirmations should be positive, present-tense, and specific, addressing areas where you seek growth and empowerment. By focusing on affirmations that truly reflect your values and goals, you can create a powerful tool for personal transformation.

Incorporating affirmations into your daily life is essential for their effectiveness. Integrate affirmations into your routine, such as repeating them during meditation, writing them in a journal, or placing them in visible locations around your home. By making affirmations a regular part of your day, you reinforce their positive messages and strengthen your commitment to self-growth.

August 8
- **Affirmation:** "I am confident in my unique talents and abilities."
- **Reflection:** "Your unique talents and abilities make you special and valuable."
- **Practical Exercise:** List your unique talents and abilities. Reflect on how you can use these strengths to achieve your goals.

August 9
- **Affirmation:** "I deserve to feel confident and self-assured."
- **Reflection:** "Confidence comes from recognizing and embracing your worth."
- **Practical Exercise:** Stand in front of a mirror and say positive affirmations to yourself. Notice how it feels to affirm your worth and confidence.

August 10

- **Affirmation:** "I will focus on my strengths and positive qualities."
- **Reflection:** "Focusing on your strengths helps build a positive self-image."
- **Practical Exercise:** Write about your strengths and positive qualities. Reflect on how these attributes have helped you in the past and how they can continue to support you.

August 11

- **Affirmation:** "I will recognize and challenge my negative self-talk."
- **Reflection:** "Challenging negative self-talk is essential for building self-esteem."
- **Practical Exercise:** Keep a journal of negative self-talk throughout the day. Reflect on each instance and write a positive counter-statement.

August 12

- **Affirmation:** "I will not compare myself to others; I am unique and valuable."
- **Reflection:** "Comparison is detrimental to self-esteem. Embrace your uniqueness."
- **Practical Exercise:** Reflect on areas where you compare yourself to others. Write about your unique qualities and why they are valuable.

August 13

- **Affirmation:** "I can learn from my mistakes and grow stronger."
- **Reflection:** "Mistakes are opportunities for growth, not reflections of your worth."
- **Practical Exercise:** Write about a recent mistake and what you learned from it. Reflect on how this lesson can help you grow.

August 14

- **Affirmation:** "I will forgive myself for past mistakes and move forward."

- **Reflection:** "Self-forgiveness is crucial for rebuilding self-esteem."
- **Practical Exercise:** Write a letter to yourself, forgiving past mistakes and offering encouragement for the future.

Week 3: Overcoming Negative Self-Perceptions

Negative self-perceptions can profoundly impact your self-esteem, affecting how you view yourself and interact with the world. These harmful thoughts often stem from past experiences, societal pressures, or internalized criticism and can create a distorted image of your true self. Understanding and dismantling these negative self-perceptions is key to replacing them with healthier and more positive self-views.

Examples of Negative Self-Perceptions

- "I am not good enough."
- "I always fail at everything I try."
- "I don't deserve to be happy."
- "I am unlovable."
- "I am a burden to others."
- "I am unattractive."
- "I am not smart enough."
- "I can't do anything right."
- "I am worthless."
- "I am a disappointment."
- "I am too weak to handle challenges."
- "I don't fit in anywhere."
- "I am incapable of success."
- "I am always the problem."
- "I am inferior to others."

Understanding the roots of negative self-perceptions is the first step toward overcoming them. These perceptions often begin in childhood and are influenced by family dynamics, educational experiences, and peer interactions. As you grow, these early influences can solidify into persistent negative beliefs about yourself. Recognizing the origins of these perceptions can help you understand that they are not intrinsic truths but learned patterns of thinking.

Identify the specific negative self-perceptions that undermine your self-esteem. Pay close attention to your inner dialogue and notice the critical or self-deprecating thoughts that arise. By bringing these thoughts to the forefront, you can begin to challenge their validity and understand the impact they have on your self-worth.

Challenging negative self-perceptions requires a conscious effort to confront and question their accuracy. Techniques such as cognitive restructuring involve re-evaluating negative thoughts and replacing them with more balanced and realistic perspectives. This process helps to weaken the hold of negative perceptions and fosters a more positive and compassionate self-view.

Developing healthier self-perceptions also involves cultivating self-compassion and self-acceptance. This means treating yourself with the same kindness and understanding that you would offer a friend. By practicing self-compassion, you can counteract the harsh self-criticism that fuels negative self-perceptions and begin to build a foundation of self-love and acceptance.

Positive affirmations can reprogram your mind to focus on your strengths and achievements rather than your perceived flaws. By consistently affirming your worth and capabilities, you can reinforce positive self-perceptions and boost your overall self-esteem.

August 15
- **Affirmation:** "I will focus on my progress, not my perfection."
- **Reflection:** "Progress, not perfection, is the key to

building self-esteem."
- **Practical Exercise:** Reflect on your progress in a specific area of your life. Write about how focusing on progress rather than perfection impacts your self-esteem.

August 16
- **Affirmation:** "I will embrace my imperfections as part of my uniqueness."
- **Reflection:** "Imperfections make you unique and human."
- **Practical Exercise:** Write about your perceived imperfections and how they contribute to your uniqueness. Reflect on why embracing them is important for self-acceptance.

August 17
- **Affirmation:** "I will practice self-love and nurture my self-esteem."
- **Reflection:** "Self-love is essential for a healthy self-image."
- **Practical Exercise:** Engage in an activity that makes you feel loved and nurtured. Reflect on how this activity enhances your self-esteem.

August 18
- **Affirmation:** "I will surround myself with positive influences that uplift me."
- **Reflection:** "Positive influences help reinforce a healthy self-image."
- **Practical Exercise:** Identify positive influences in your life (people, activities, environments). Make a plan to spend more time engaging with these influences.

August 19
- **Affirmation:** "I will practice gratitude for who I am and what I have."
- **Reflection:** "Gratitude fosters a positive mindset and self-image."
- **Practical Exercise:** Write a gratitude list focusing on qualities and achievements you appreciate about

yourself. Reflect on how practicing gratitude impacts your self-esteem.

August 20
- **Affirmation:** "I will celebrate my individuality and unique qualities."
- **Reflection:** "Celebrating your individuality enhances your self-worth."
- **Practical Exercise:** Reflect on what makes you unique. Write a list of qualities that set you apart and why you value them.

August 21
- **Affirmation:** "I am committed to my journey of self-esteem and self-worth."
- **Reflection:** "Commitment to your self-esteem journey is crucial for long-term growth."
- **Practical Exercise:** Write a commitment statement to yourself about maintaining and enhancing your self-esteem. Reflect on the steps you will take to honor this commitment.

Week 4: Building a Positive Self-Image

Building a positive self-image involves embracing who you are, recognizing your inherent worth, and fostering a mindset that supports self-acceptance and growth. Various techniques and practices can help you cultivate and maintain a positive self-image over time. Understanding that self-image is not static, but a dynamic and evolving perception is crucial in this journey.

The foundations of a positive self-image emphasize the importance of self-awareness and self-acceptance. Recognizing your strengths, achievements, and unique qualities forms the bedrock of a healthy self-image. Engage in exercises that help you identify and celebrate these aspects of yourself, reinforcing the understanding that you are worthy and valuable just as you are.

The role of self-talk significantly influences how you perceive yourself. Negative self-talk can undermine your self-esteem, while positive affirmations can boost your confidence and self-worth. Practice transforming negative self-talk into positive affirmations, helping you develop a more supportive and compassionate inner dialogue.

External influences can contribute to a distorted self-perception. By critically evaluating these influences and setting boundaries, you can protect and nurture your self-image. Strategies to minimize the impact of negative external feedback and focus on sources of positive reinforcement are essential.

Self-compassion is crucial in building a positive self-image. Being kind to yourself during moments of failure or imperfection is essential for maintaining a healthy self-image. Practice self-compassion exercises that encourage you to treat yourself with the same kindness and understanding you would offer a close friend, fostering resilience and emotional well-being.

Setting and achieving personal goals reinforces your belief in your capabilities and contributes to a sense of purpose and fulfillment. Set realistic and achievable goals and create action plans to help you reach them, celebrating each step forward as a testament to your growth and potential.

Mindfulness and gratitude enhance your self-image. Mindfulness helps you stay present and appreciate the moment, reducing the tendency to dwell on past mistakes or worry about the future. Practicing gratitude shifts your focus to the positive aspects of your life and yourself, reinforcing a positive self-image. Incorporate mindfulness and gratitude exercises into your daily routine, helping you maintain a balanced and appreciative perspective on yourself and your life.

August 22

- **Affirmation:** "I will set boundaries to protect my self-esteem."
- **Reflection:** "Boundaries are essential for maintaining a healthy self-image."
- **Practical Exercise:** Identify a situation where setting a boundary could protect your self-esteem. Plan and practice how you will assert this boundary.

August 23

- **Affirmation:** "I will seek support from those who uplift and encourage me."
- **Reflection:** "Supportive relationships are vital for sustaining self-esteem."
- **Practical Exercise:** Reach out to a supportive friend or mentor. Share your journey and seek their encouragement and support.

August 24

- **Affirmation:** "I will practice self-reflection to continue growing."
- **Reflection:** "Self-reflection helps you stay aware of your progress and areas for growth."
- **Practical Exercise:** Set aside time for self-reflection. Write about your self-esteem journey, noting progress and areas where you can continue to grow.

August 25

- **Affirmation:** "I will celebrate my successes and learn from my challenges."
- **Reflection:** "Celebrating successes and learning from challenges fosters resilience and growth."
- **Practical Exercise:** Reflect on recent successes and challenges. Write about what you learned from each and how they contribute to your self-esteem.

August 26

- **Affirmation:** "I will nurture my self-esteem with positive self-talk and affirmations."
- **Reflection:** "Positive self-talk reinforces a healthy self-

image."

- **Practical Exercise:** Create a list of positive affirmations that resonate with you. Repeat them daily and reflect on their impact on your self-esteem.

August 27

- **Affirmation:** "I will engage in activities that align with my values and passions."
- **Reflection:** "Pursuing activities that align with your values enhances your sense of self-worth."
- **Practical Exercise:** Identify an activity that aligns with your values and passions. Plan to engage in this activity regularly and reflect on its impact on your self-esteem.

August 28

- **Affirmation:** "I will practice self-care to support my mental and emotional well-being."
- **Reflection:** "Self-care is fundamental for maintaining self-esteem."
- **Practical Exercise:** Create a self-care routine that includes activities that nurture your mind, body, and spirit. Reflect on how this routine supports your self-esteem.

August 29

- **Affirmation:** "I will embrace change as an opportunity for growth."
- **Reflection:** "Embracing change helps you adapt and grow stronger."
- **Practical Exercise:** Reflect on a recent change in your life. Write about how you can view this change as an opportunity for growth and self-improvement.

August 30

- **Affirmation:** "I am proud of my journey and the person I am becoming."
- **Reflection:** "Pride in your journey reinforces a positive self-image."
- **Practical Exercise:** Write about your self-esteem journey over the past month. Reflect on the progress

you have made and celebrate your achievements.

August 31
- **Affirmation:** "I am committed to nurturing my self-esteem and living authentically."
- **Reflection:** "Authenticity and self-esteem go hand in hand."
- **Practical Exercise:** Reflect on what living authentically means to you. Write about how you will continue to nurture your self-esteem by embracing your authentic self.

August Conclusion

As we conclude this month dedicated to rebuilding self-esteem, take a moment to reflect deeply on the significant progress you have made. Recognizing your worth, challenging negative self-perceptions, and embracing a positive self-image are pivotal steps in this transformative journey. Rebuilding self-esteem is not a destination but an ongoing process that demands dedication, self-compassion, and consistent effort.

Understanding and recognizing your inherent worth has laid a strong foundation for your self-esteem. By appreciating your unique qualities, strengths, and contributions, you have begun to see yourself in a new light, less reliant on external validation and more confident in your intrinsic value.

Positive affirmations have played a crucial role in reshaping your thoughts and beliefs. By consistently reinforcing positive self-perceptions, you have worked to replace negative self-talk with empowering messages. This practice has helped you build a more supportive and nurturing inner dialogue, boosting your confidence and self-worth.

Overcoming negative self-perceptions has been a key focus this month. By identifying and challenging the harmful thoughts and beliefs that have undermined your self-esteem, you have taken significant steps toward a healthier self-image. Through cognitive restructuring and self-compassion, you have begun to dismantle these distortions and cultivate a more balanced and realistic view of yourself.

Building a positive self-image involves embracing who you are, setting and achieving personal goals, and fostering a mindset that supports self-acceptance and growth. By celebrating your individuality and unique qualities, you have reinforced your belief in your capabilities and developed a sense of purpose and fulfillment. Incorporating mindfulness and gratitude into your daily routine has further enhanced your self-image, helping you maintain a balanced and appreciative perspective on yourself and your life.

Throughout this month, you have diligently practiced self-reflection, engaged in activities that resonate with your values and passions, and surrounded yourself with positive influences. These practices are essential in enhancing your self-worth and fostering a healthy self-esteem. Remember, the foundation of self-esteem lies in the understanding that you are deserving of love, respect, and kindness, both from yourself and others.

Reflect on the skills you have acquired and the insights you have gained. By identifying and challenging negative thoughts, you have learned to replace them with empowering beliefs. This shift in perspective is crucial for maintaining a positive self-image. You have also discovered the importance of setting and achieving personal goals, which reinforces your sense of accomplishment and self-worth.

Celebrate the milestones you have reached and the resilience you have shown. Each step forward, no matter how small, is a testament to your strength and determination. Acknowledge the moments when you chose to prioritize your well-being and recognize the courage it takes to face and overcome self-doubt. These victories, both big and small, are significant markers on your path to a more positive and fulfilling life.

As you move forward, continue to nurture your self-esteem with the tools and practices you have learned this month. Consistency is key to maintaining the progress you have made. Revisit your affirmations, engage in regular self-reflection, and immerse yourself in activities that bring you joy and fulfillment. Surround yourself with supportive individuals who uplift and encourage you.

Remember, the journey of self-esteem is ongoing. Each day is an opportunity to reaffirm your worth and celebrate your unique qualities. Keep moving forward with confidence and self-compassion, knowing that every step you take brings you closer to a life filled with positivity and self-love. You are deserving of all the good that life has to offer, and your journey toward self-esteem is a powerful testament to your incredible potential.

September: Creating a Support System

Creating a strong support system is essential for your mental, emotional, and overall well-being. This month, we will explore the importance of supportive relationships, identify potential sources of support, and develop strategies to build and maintain a robust support network. A well-rounded support system can provide the comfort, guidance, and encouragement you need as you navigate life's challenges. By the end of this month, you will be equipped with the tools and knowledge to create a network that empowers you to thrive.

Support systems are crucial in helping you cope with stress, make important decisions, and stay motivated during difficult times. They offer a sense of belonging and security, reminding you that you are not alone in your journey. Whether it's family, friends, mentors, or professional counselors, having a variety of supportive people in your life can significantly impact your resilience and overall happiness. This month, we will explore how to identify and nurture these essential connections.

Identifying potential sources of support involves looking at the various people in your life who can offer different types of assistance. This might include emotional support from friends and family, practical support from colleagues and mentors, and professional support from therapists and counselors. We will guide you in evaluating your current relationships and recognizing where there might be gaps in your support network. By doing so, you can better understand where to seek new connections or strengthen existing ones.

Building a support system requires intentional effort and communication. It's about being open to giving and receiving help, establishing trust, and setting healthy boundaries. This month, you will learn strategies for effectively communicating your needs and expectations with those in your support network. Additionally, we will discuss how to offer support to others, creating a reciprocal and mutually beneficial relationship.

Maintaining a support system is an ongoing process. Relationships need to be nurtured and regularly attended to in order to remain strong and effective. You will discover techniques for staying connected with your support network, such as regular check-ins, shared activities, and showing appreciation for their presence in your life. We will also address common challenges in maintaining a support network, such as dealing with conflicts and balancing your needs with those of others.

Week 1: Identifying Supportive Individuals

Introduction of Week's Theme

Identifying individuals who can provide genuine support is the first step in building a robust support system, essential for navigating life's challenges and fostering personal growth. This week, we will focus on recognizing the qualities of supportive people, identifying those in your life who embody these traits, and understanding how to cultivate and maintain these valuable relationships. By the end of this week, you will have a clearer understanding of who in your life can truly offer the support you need and how to strengthen these connections.

Supportive individuals build you up, support you, trust you, have your back, accept you, and do not judge you. Supportive individuals often exhibit specific qualities that make them reliable and trustworthy allies. These qualities include empathy, active listening, reliability, and non-judgmental attitudes. Empathy allows them to understand and share your feelings, making you feel seen and heard. Active listening involves giving you their full attention and responding thoughtfully, showing that they genuinely care about what you have to say. Reliability means they can be counted on to be there for you consistently. At the same time, a non-judgmental attitude ensures you can share your thoughts and feelings without fear of criticism or rejection.

Recognizing these qualities in the people around you is crucial for building a strong support network. Start by reflecting on your interactions with friends, family, and colleagues. Who listens without interrupting? Who offers comfort and understanding without passing judgment? Who can you count on to be there for you during tough times? These are the people who can provide the foundation of your support system.

In addition to identifying supportive individuals, it's important to understand the dynamics of your relationships. Some people in your life may not be inherently unsupportive but might lack the skills or awareness to provide the support you need. In such cases, communication is key. Openly discussing your needs and how they can help can strengthen these relationships and transform them into sources of genuine support. Be clear about what you need—whether it's a listening ear, practical help, or emotional encouragement—and give them the opportunity to step up.

Remember, identifying and cultivating supportive relationships is not just about seeking help when needed but also about creating a balanced, reciprocal network where you, too, offer support and understanding. This mutual exchange strengthens bonds and fosters a sense of community and belonging. As you progress through this week, keep in mind that support is a two-way street, and by being a supportive friend or family member yourself, you contribute to a healthier, more resilient network.

September 1

- **Affirmation:** "I deserve to be surrounded by supportive and caring individuals."
- **Reflection:** "Supportive relationships are vital for your well-being."
- **Practical Exercise:** Make a list of qualities that define a supportive person (e.g., empathy, reliability, positivity). Reflect on individuals in your life who possess these qualities.

September 2

- **Affirmation:** "I will seek out relationships that uplift and encourage me."
- **Reflection:** "Positive relationships enhance your mental and emotional health."
- **Practical Exercise:** Identify three people in your life who uplift and encourage you. Plan to reach out to them this week to strengthen your connection.

September 3

- **Affirmation:** "I can recognize and appreciate those who support me."
- **Reflection:** "Acknowledging supportive people strengthens your bond with them."
- **Practical Exercise:** Write a note of appreciation to someone who has been supportive of you. Reflect on how expressing gratitude enhances your relationship.

September 4

- **Affirmation:** "I will prioritize relationships that contribute to my growth and happiness."
- **Reflection:** "Investing in positive relationships supports your overall well-being."
- **Practical Exercise:** Reflect on your current relationships and identify which ones contribute to your growth and happiness. Plan to spend more time nurturing these connections.

September 5

- **Affirmation:** "I am open to building new supportive relationships."
- **Reflection:** "Being open to new connections can expand your support network."
- **Practical Exercise:** Attend a social event or join a group activity to meet new people. Reflect on how these new connections can support you.

September 6

- **Affirmation:** "I will build trust by being reliable and honest."
- **Reflection:** "Reliability and honesty are key components of trust."
- **Practical Exercise:** Reflect on how you can demonstrate reliability and honesty in your relationships. Make a plan to practice these qualities consistently.

September 7

- **Affirmation:** "I will communicate openly to build trust with others."
- **Reflection:** "Open communication fosters trust and understanding."
- **Practical Exercise:** Practice open communication with a trusted friend or family member. Share something meaningful and encourage them to do the same.

Week 2: Building Trusting Relationships

Introduction of Week's Theme

Building trust is a fundamental aspect of creating a strong support system. Trust serves as the cornerstone of healthy, fulfilling relationships, fostering a sense of security and reliability that allows individuals to feel supported and understood. This week, we will explore the multifaceted nature of trust, exploring its importance, how it is built, and strategies to maintain it over time.

Trust begins with authenticity and transparency. Being genuine in your interactions and open about your thoughts and feelings lays the groundwork for others to feel comfortable and secure in your relationship. It involves being honest, even when the truth is difficult, and ensuring that your words align with your actions. This consistency between what you say and what you do helps to establish a reliable foundation on which trust can be built.

Another crucial element in building trust is active listening. When you listen attentively and empathetically, you validate the other person's experiences and emotions. This creates a safe space for open communication where both parties feel heard and respected. Active listening also involves being present in the moment, showing interest through body language, and refraining from interrupting or judging.

Mutual respect is also integral to developing trust. This means acknowledging and valuing each other's boundaries, opinions, and differences. Respecting boundaries shows that you care about the other person's comfort and well-being, which in turn fosters trust. It is essential to communicate openly about your boundaries and listen to those of others, ensuring that both parties feel respected and secure.

Accountability plays a significant role in maintaining trust. Taking responsibility for your actions, admitting when you are wrong, and making amends where necessary demonstrate integrity and reliability. This willingness to be accountable shows that you are committed to the relationship and willing to put in the effort to maintain trust. It also encourages the other person to do the same, creating a reciprocal dynamic of trust and accountability.

Consistency is key in sustaining trust over time. Regularly demonstrating trustworthy behavior reinforces the foundation of trust you have built. This involves keeping promises, being dependable, and showing up for the other person consistently. Over time, these consistent actions reinforce the belief that you are reliable and trustworthy, further strengthening the bond.

September 8

- **Affirmation:** "I will respect others' boundaries to build mutual trust."
- **Reflection:** "Respecting boundaries is essential for maintaining trust."
- **Practical Exercise:** Reflect on the boundaries of those in your support system. Make a conscious effort to respect these boundaries and discuss your own.

September 9

- **Affirmation:** "I can rebuild trust if it has been broken."
- **Reflection:** "Rebuilding trust takes time and effort but is possible."
- **Practical Exercise:** Identify a relationship where trust has been broken. Reflect on steps you can take to rebuild trust, such as apologizing or making amends.

September 10

- **Affirmation:** "I will be patient in building trusting relationships."
- **Reflection:** "Trust develops over time with consistent effort."
- **Practical Exercise:** Reflect on the importance of patience in building trust. Write about how you can practice patience in your relationships.

September 11

- **Affirmation:** "I will invest time and energy into my friendships."
- **Reflection:** "Quality friendships require dedication and effort."
- **Practical Exercise:** Plan a meaningful activity with a friend this week. Reflect on how spending quality time together strengthens your bond.

September 12
  - **Affirmation:** "I will communicate my appreciation to my friends."
  - **Reflection:** "Expressing appreciation fosters positive relationships."
  - **Practical Exercise:** Write a message of appreciation to a friend, expressing why you value their friendship. Reflect on how this gesture impacts your relationship.

September 13
  - **Affirmation:** "I will listen actively and empathetically to my friends."
  - **Reflection:** "Active listening shows you value and respect your friends' experiences."
  - **Practical Exercise:** Practice active listening in a conversation with a friend. Reflect on how this deepens your connection and understanding.

September 14
  - **Affirmation:** "I will support my friends in their times of need."
  - **Reflection:** "Being there for your friends strengthens your mutual support."
  - **Practical Exercise:** Identify a friend who may need support and reach out to offer your help. Reflect on how this act of kindness strengthens your friendship.

Week 3: Nurturing Healthy Friendships

Introduction of Week's Theme

Nurturing healthy friendships is an essential aspect of building a fulfilling and supportive social network. Healthy friendships contribute significantly to our emotional well-being, providing us with a sense of belonging, support, and mutual understanding. This week, we will explore the nuances of cultivating and maintaining strong friendships, ensuring that they remain positive and enriching aspects of our lives.

Developing and maintaining healthy friendships requires

ongoing effort and intentionality. It's not just about finding friends but also about actively nurturing these relationships to ensure they thrive. Healthy friendships are characterized by mutual respect, trust, and open communication. This week, we will explore practical strategies for enhancing these elements in your friendships, helping you build deeper and more meaningful connections.

Effective communication is the cornerstone of any healthy relationship. This includes not only speaking honestly and openly but also listening actively and empathetically. We will discuss techniques for improving your communication skills, such as active listening, expressing appreciation, and providing constructive feedback. By fostering open lines of communication, you can ensure that your friendships are based on mutual understanding and respect.

Trust is another vital component of strong friendships. Building trust involves being reliable, keeping confidence, and showing up for your friends in times of need. This week, we will explore ways to build and maintain trust in your friendships. We will also address how to rebuild trust if it has been broken, ensuring that your relationships remain resilient and enduring.

Supportive friendships are those where both parties feel valued and cared for. This means offering emotional support during difficult times and celebrating each other's successes. We will discuss how to be a supportive friend, including recognizing when your friends need support, offering help, and being present. By being a supportive friend, you can strengthen your relationships and create a network of people who are there for you when you need them.

Boundaries are essential in any healthy relationship, including friendships. Setting and respecting boundaries ensures that both parties feel comfortable and respected. This week, we will explore how to establish healthy boundaries in your friendships and communicate them effectively. Understanding and respecting each other's boundaries can prevent misunderstandings and foster a sense of mutual respect.

Nurturing healthy friendships involves mutual effort and commitment. Friendships require regular attention and care to flourish. We will discuss practical ways to nurture your friendships, such as spending quality time together, engaging in shared activities, and expressing gratitude. By making an intentional effort to nurture your friendships, you can ensure that they remain a positive and supportive part of your life.

September 15
- **Affirmation:** "I will set healthy boundaries to maintain balanced friendships."
- **Reflection:** "Healthy boundaries ensure mutual respect and balance in friendships."
- **Practical Exercise:** Reflect on the boundaries within your friendships. Communicate any necessary boundaries to your friends to ensure mutual understanding.

September 16
- **Affirmation:** "I will communicate openly and honestly with my friends."
- **Reflection:** "Open and honest communication is the foundation of a strong friendship."
- **Practical Exercise:** Practice active listening and share your thoughts and feelings openly with a close friend. Notice how this deepens your connection.

September 17
- **Affirmation:** "I will be reliable and trustworthy in my friendships."
- **Reflection:** "Being dependable builds trust and strengthens friendships."
- **Practical Exercise:** Reflect on how you can be more reliable in your friendships. Make a commitment to follow through on your promises.

September 18

- **Affirmation:** "I will offer support and celebrate my friends' successes."
- **Reflection:** "Supporting your friends and celebrating their achievements fosters a positive relationship."
- **Practical Exercise:** Reach out to a friend to offer support or celebrate a recent success. Reflect on how this strengthens your bond.

September 19

- **Affirmation:** "I will respect my friends' boundaries and communicate my own."
- **Reflection:** "Mutual respect for boundaries is crucial for healthy friendships."
- **Practical Exercise:** Identify and communicate a personal boundary to a friend. Reflect on how respecting each other's boundaries enhances your friendship.

September 20

- **Affirmation:** "I will make time to nurture my friendships."
- **Reflection:** "Regular attention and care are essential for maintaining strong friendships."
- **Practical Exercise:** Schedule a regular activity or meeting with a friend. Reflect on how spending quality time together nurtures your relationship.

September 21

- **Affirmation:** "I will express gratitude for my friends and the support they provide."
- **Reflection:** "Expressing gratitude strengthens bonds and fosters a positive environment."
- **Practical Exercise:** Write a heartfelt note or message to a friend expressing your gratitude for their friendship. Reflect on the impact of this gesture on your relationship.

Week 4: Sustaining and Strengthening

Your Support System

Introduction of Week's Theme

Maintaining and strengthening your support system is an ongoing process that requires attention and care. A strong support network can significantly impact your mental health and overall well-being by providing emotional support, practical help, and a sense of belonging. This week, we will explore various strategies to sustain and enhance your support network, ensuring that you have a reliable and nurturing community around you.

First, it's essential to understand the different components that make up a robust support system. Your network can include family members, friends, colleagues, mentors, and even professional support such as therapists or counselors. Each of these connections plays a unique role in providing support, and recognizing these roles can help you better appreciate and cultivate your relationships.

Regular communication is a cornerstone of maintaining strong relationships. This involves more than just staying in touch; it means engaging in meaningful conversations, being present, and showing genuine interest in the lives of those in your support system. This week, we will explore techniques for effective communication, including active listening, expressing gratitude, and offering support in return.

Another critical aspect of a healthy support system is mutual respect and understanding. Building and maintaining trust requires transparency, reliability, and empathy. We will explore ways to foster trust and respect in your relationships, addressing conflicts constructively and ensuring that your connections are based on mutual care and understanding.

In addition to nurturing existing relationships, expanding your support network is also beneficial. This can involve reaching out to new people, joining groups or communities with shared interests, and seeking out new professional support if needed. Diversifying your support system can provide you with a broader range of perspectives and resources.

Self-care and boundaries are also crucial in maintaining a healthy support network. It's important to recognize your limits and communicate them clearly to prevent burnout and ensure that your support system remains a positive influence in your life. We will discuss strategies for setting and maintaining healthy boundaries within your relationships.

By the end of this week, you will have a deeper understanding of the importance of a strong support network and the tools to maintain and enhance it effectively. Remember, building and sustaining a supportive community is a dynamic process that evolves with time. Stay committed to nurturing your relationships, and you will reap the benefits of a solid support system that enriches your life and supports your journey toward well-being.

September 22
- **Affirmation:** "I will be mindful of the support I give and receive."
- **Reflection:** "Balance in giving and receiving support is crucial for healthy relationships."
- **Practical Exercise:** Reflect on the balance of support in your relationships. Write about how you can ensure mutual support and maintain this balance.

September 23
- **Affirmation:** "I will adapt my support system as my needs evolve."
- **Reflection:** "Your support needs may change over time, and your support system should adapt accordingly."
- **Practical Exercise:** Reflect on your current support needs and how they have changed. Write about any adjustments you need to make to your support system.

September 24

- **Affirmation:** "I will nurture my support system with care and attention."
- **Reflection:** "Ongoing care and attention help sustain strong support networks."
- **Practical Exercise:** Identify ways to nurture your support system (e.g., regular gatherings, expressions of gratitude). Implement one of these ideas this week.

September 25

- **Affirmation:** "I will seek feedback from my support system to improve our relationships."
- **Reflection:** "Feedback helps you understand and strengthen your relationships."
- **Practical Exercise:** Ask a trusted member of your support system for feedback on your relationship. Reflect on their insights and how you can use them to improve your connection.

September 26

- **Affirmation:** "I will be flexible and open to changes within my support system."
- **Reflection:** "Flexibility and openness ensure your support system remains effective and relevant."
- **Practical Exercise:** Reflect on recent changes within your support system. Write about how you can be more flexible and open to these changes.

September 27

- **Affirmation:** "I will celebrate the strength and resilience of my support system."
- **Reflection:** "Celebrating your support system reinforces its importance and value."
- **Practical Exercise:** Plan a small celebration or gathering to honor the members of your support system. Reflect on how this celebration strengthens your connections.

September 28

- **Affirmation:** "I am grateful for the support I receive

and the relationships I have built."
  - **Reflection:** "Gratitude fosters a positive mindset and reinforces the value of your support system."
  - **Practical Exercise:** Write a gratitude list focusing on the support you have received and the relationships you have built. Reflect on how gratitude enhances your well-being.

September 29
  - **Affirmation:** "I will continue to invest in my support system for my well-being."
  - **Reflection:** "Ongoing investment in your support system is crucial for long-term well-being."
  - **Practical Exercise:** Reflect on how you can continue to invest in your support system. Write about specific actions you will take to maintain and strengthen your network.

September 30
  - **Affirmation:** "I am committed to fostering a strong and supportive community."
  - **Reflection:** "A strong and supportive community contributes to your overall happiness and resilience."
  - **Practical Exercise:** Write a commitment statement about your role in fostering a strong and supportive community. Reflect on the steps you will take to honor this commitment.

September Conclusion

Identifying supportive individuals, building trusting relationships, and nurturing healthy friendships are critical components of developing a strong support network. This process is ongoing and requires continuous dedication, open communication, and mutual respect. By recognizing the importance of these elements, you have laid a solid foundation for a resilient support system.

You have explored the various aspects of seeking professional support, maintaining regular contact with your support system, and adapting to changing needs. These steps have strengthened your current support network and empowered you to navigate future challenges with greater confidence. Your willingness to reach out for help and offer support in return has created a cycle of positivity and resilience.

Building a support network is a continuous journey. Each interaction, conversation, and act of kindness contributes to the growth and strength of your support system. Celebrate the progress you've made and acknowledge the efforts you've put into fostering these connections. This reinforces the value of these relationships and motivates you to continue nurturing them.

Maintaining regular contact with your support system shows your commitment to both giving and receiving support. This reciprocal dynamic is crucial in creating a balanced and sustainable network. Your adaptability in meeting your and others' changing needs demonstrates a deep understanding of the fluid nature of relationships and the importance of flexibility in maintaining them.

As you move forward, continue to invest time and energy into your support system. Celebrate the small victories and milestones along the way, and remember that each step you take brings you closer to a stronger and more supportive community. A robust support network is a valuable resource that can help you navigate life's ups and downs with greater ease and confidence.

October: Forgiveness and Letting Go

Forgiveness and letting go are fundamental steps in the healing process, essential for overcoming past hurts and moving forward with your life. This month, we will explore understanding the process of forgiveness and exploring its profound impact on your emotional and mental well-being. We will examine the benefits of letting go, recognizing how holding onto pain and resentment can hinder your growth and happiness. By learning to release these burdens, you can find inner peace, improve your relationships, and open up new avenues for personal development.

Forgiveness is often misunderstood as condoning or excusing harmful behavior, but it is actually a powerful act of self-liberation. It involves acknowledging the pain inflicted upon you, accepting that you cannot change the past, and choosing to release the hold that this pain has on your life. This month, we will focus on breaking down the process of forgiveness into manageable steps, making it accessible and achievable. You will learn that forgiveness is not about the offender but about your own healing and empowerment.

Letting go is another crucial aspect of emotional freedom. Holding onto grudges, anger, and resentment can weigh heavily on your heart and mind, affecting your daily life and overall well-being. We will explore the detrimental effects of clinging to past hurts and how letting go can lighten your emotional load. By understanding the importance of letting go, you can begin to free yourself from the chains of past traumas and negative experiences, paving the way for a more positive and fulfilling life.

As we embark on this journey of forgiveness and letting go, it is important to remember that this process takes time and patience. Healing is not linear, and you may encounter setbacks along the way. However, each step you take toward forgiveness and letting go brings you closer to inner peace and emotional freedom. Embrace this month as an opportunity to release the past and make room for new experiences, growth, and happiness. Together, we will work toward a brighter future, one where you are no longer held back by the pain of the past but empowered to live your life to the fullest.

Week 1: Understanding Forgiveness

Introduction of Week's Theme

Forgiveness is a multifaceted and deeply personal process that encompasses releasing resentment, letting go of grudges, and moving toward emotional freedom. This week, we will explore the concept of forgiveness, exploring its nuances, benefits, and the steps required to embark on this transformative journey. Understanding forgiveness is crucial for personal growth, as it allows you to heal from past wounds and cultivate a more peaceful and fulfilling life.

Forgiveness is often misunderstood as condoning or excusing harmful behavior. However, true forgiveness is about acknowledging the hurt, holding those responsible accountable, and making a conscious decision to let go of the anger and resentment that bind you to the past. It's a process that involves self-reflection, empathy, and a commitment to your own healing. By understanding the true essence of forgiveness, you can begin to see it as a powerful tool for liberation rather than a sign of weakness or surrender.

The benefits of forgiveness extend beyond emotional relief. Studies have shown that forgiving others can lead to improved mental and physical health, stronger relationships, and a greater sense of well-being. By letting go of grudges, you free yourself from the negative emotions that can drain your energy and cloud your judgment. This week, we will explore these benefits in depth, helping you to see how forgiveness can be a gift you give yourself.

Forgiving others can be challenging, especially when the hurt is deep and the wounds are fresh. It requires empathy and understanding, allowing you to see the situation from the perspective of the person who hurt you. This doesn't mean justifying their actions but rather recognizing their humanity and imperfections. We will discuss strategies to develop empathy and compassion, which are essential components of the forgiveness process.

Self-forgiveness is equally important and often more difficult to achieve. Holding onto guilt and self-blame can hinder your personal growth and prevent you from moving forward. This week, we will explore the steps to forgive yourself for past mistakes, understanding that self-compassion is a crucial part of the healing process. By forgiving yourself, you acknowledge your own humanity and allow yourself the grace to learn and grow from your experiences.

Beginning the journey of forgiveness involves practical steps and a supportive mindset. We will provide exercises and reflections to help you identify whom you need to forgive, including yourself, and outline the steps to start this journey. These activities will guide you through acknowledging your pain, expressing your feelings, and gradually letting go of the negative emotions that hold you back. Through these exercises, you will gain clarity and strength to embrace forgiveness as a path to inner peace and emotional freedom.

As we embark on this week dedicated to understanding forgiveness, remember that this process is a journey, not a destination. It requires time, patience, and persistence. Celebrate small victories and be gentle with yourself as you navigate through your emotions. The goal is not to forget the past but to free yourself from its hold, allowing you to live more fully in the present. Together, let's explore the power of forgiveness and how it can transform your life.

October 1

- **Affirmation:** "I am open to understanding the true meaning of forgiveness."
- **Reflection:** "Forgiveness is about releasing resentment, not condoning hurtful behavior."
- **Practical Exercise:** Reflect on the concept of forgiveness. Write about what forgiveness means to you and how it can benefit your life.

October 2

- **Affirmation:** "Forgiveness is a gift I give to myself."
- **Reflection:** "Forgiveness frees you from the burden of resentment and anger."
- **Practical Exercise:** Identify a situation where you have been holding onto resentment. Reflect on how forgiving the person involved can benefit your emotional well-being.

October 3

- **Affirmation:** "I can choose to forgive and let go of past hurts."
- **Reflection:** "Forgiveness is a choice and a powerful step toward healing."
- **Practical Exercise:** Write about a past hurt you are willing to forgive. Reflect on the steps you need to take to begin the process of forgiveness.

October 4

- **Affirmation:** "I will practice self-compassion as I work through forgiveness."

- **Reflection:** "Being kind to yourself is crucial when working through difficult emotions."
- **Practical Exercise:** Write a letter to yourself offering compassion and understanding as you navigate the process of forgiveness.

October 5

- **Affirmation:** "I release the need for revenge and embrace the power of forgiveness."
- **Reflection:** "Letting go of the desire for revenge allows you to move forward."
- **Practical Exercise:** Reflect on any feelings of revenge you may have. Write about how releasing these feelings can lead to a more peaceful and fulfilling life.

October 6

- **Affirmation:** "Forgiveness is a journey, and I am committed to it."
- **Reflection:** "Commitment to the process of forgiveness can bring lasting peace."
- **Practical Exercise:** Identify the steps you are willing to take to commit to forgiveness. Write them down and revisit them regularly.

October 7

- **Affirmation:** "I am patient with myself as I learn to forgive."
- **Reflection:** "Forgiveness is a process that takes time and patience."
- **Practical Exercise:** Reflect on the importance of patience in the process of forgiveness. Write about how you can practice patience with yourself and others.

Week 2: Forgiving Others

Introduction of Week's Theme

Forgiving others can be one of the most challenging but liberating processes on your journey toward healing and personal growth. It requires a deep commitment to letting go of past hurts and moving forward with a sense of peace and resolution. This week, we will explore practical strategies to forgive those who have hurt you, explore the profound benefits of releasing resentment, and understand how forgiveness can transform your emotional well-being and relationships.

Forgiveness does not mean condoning or excusing harmful behavior; instead, it is about freeing yourself from the burden of anger and bitterness. Holding onto resentment can create a heavy emotional weight, impacting your mental health, physical well-being, and relationships with others. By choosing to forgive, you allow yourself to heal and create space for positive emotions and experiences to flourish in your life.

We will begin by understanding the nature of forgiveness and why it is essential for your personal growth. Forgiveness is a conscious, deliberate decision to release feelings of resentment or vengeance toward a person or group who has harmed you. It does not mean forgetting or denying the harm done, but rather, it means letting go of the negative emotions associated with the hurtful experience. This process can lead to a sense of inner peace and emotional freedom, allowing you to move forward with a lighter heart.

Throughout this week, we will explore various techniques to help you forgive others, such as reframing your perspective, practicing empathy, and engaging in self-compassion. Reframing your perspective involves looking at the situation from a different angle, understanding the context of the other person's behavior, and recognizing that holding onto anger only harms you. Practicing empathy helps you to see the humanity in others, acknowledge their flaws, and understand that everyone makes mistakes. Engaging in self-compassion allows you to be gentle with yourself as you navigate the complex emotions associated with forgiveness.

We will also discuss the importance of setting boundaries and maintaining self-respect while forgiving others. Forgiveness does not mean allowing others to continue hurting you or diminishing your self-worth. It is about protecting yourself, setting clear boundaries, and ensuring that you do not re-enter toxic dynamics. By establishing healthy boundaries, you create a safe space for yourself to heal and grow while maintaining your dignity and self-respect.

Lastly, we will focus on the transformative power of forgiveness and how it can positively impact your life. Forgiving others can lead to improved mental health, reduced stress and anxiety, better physical health, and more fulfilling relationships. It opens the door to a more compassionate, empathetic, and joyful existence, enabling you to live a life free from the constraints of past hurts. By embracing forgiveness, you take a significant step toward personal liberation and emotional well-being.

As we embark on this week's journey, remember that forgiveness is a process that takes time and effort. Be patient with yourself, and recognize that each step you take toward forgiving others is a step toward reclaiming your peace and happiness. Let's commit to this transformative journey with open hearts and minds, knowing that the path to forgiveness is a powerful way to heal and empower yourself.

October 8
- **Affirmation:** "I am capable of forgiving those who have hurt me."
- **Reflection:** "Forgiveness is a testament to your strength and resilience."
- **Practical Exercise:** Reflect on a person you need to forgive. Write about the impact their actions have had on you and why you want to forgive them.

October 9
- **Affirmation:** "I will let go of past hurts and focus on the present."
- **Reflection:** "Letting go of the past allows you to embrace the present fully."

- **Practical Exercise:** Identify a past hurt that continues to affect you. Write about how letting go of this hurt can improve your present life.

October 10
- **Affirmation:** "I can forgive without forgetting or excusing harmful behavior."
- **Reflection:** "Forgiveness does not mean condoning or forgetting the hurtful actions."
- **Practical Exercise:** Write about how you can forgive someone while still acknowledging the harm they caused. Reflect on the balance between forgiveness and accountability.

October 11
- **Affirmation:** "I will set boundaries to protect myself while practicing forgiveness."
- **Reflection:** "Healthy boundaries are essential for maintaining your well-being."
- **Practical Exercise:** Reflect on the boundaries you need to set with someone you are forgiving. Write about how these boundaries can support your healing process.

October 12
- **Affirmation:** "I choose to forgive and release the burden of resentment."
- **Reflection:** "Releasing resentment lightens your emotional load and fosters peace."
- **Practical Exercise:** Write a letter of forgiveness to someone who has hurt you. You don't need to send it; simply writing it can be a powerful act of release.

October 13
- **Affirmation:** "I am worthy of giving and receiving forgiveness."
- **Reflection:** "Recognizing your worth is essential in the process of forgiveness."
- **Practical Exercise:** Reflect on the concept of worthiness in forgiveness. Write about why you and others deserve forgiveness.

October 14
- **Affirmation:** "I will forgive at my own pace and in my own time."
- **Reflection:** "Forgiveness is a personal journey that should be done at your own pace."
- **Practical Exercise:** Reflect on the pace at which you are comfortable with forgiving. Write about how respecting your own timeline can make the process more genuine.

Week 3: Self-Forgiveness

Introduction of Week's Theme

Self-forgiveness is a transformative and essential step in the journey toward healing and personal growth. This week, we will explore the concept of self-forgiveness, exploring its significance, the barriers that often prevent us from forgiving ourselves, and the steps we can take to cultivate a kinder, more compassionate relationship with ourselves. Recognizing the importance of self-forgiveness is crucial for breaking free from the shackles of guilt, shame, and self-criticism that often accompany experiences with toxic family dynamics.

Forgiving yourself is not about excusing or justifying past mistakes or harmful behaviors but about acknowledging them, learning from them, and allowing yourself to move forward without the heavy burden of self-blame. This process involves a profound shift in how you perceive yourself and your past actions. It requires a willingness to confront and accept your imperfections and mistakes as part of your human experience.

One of the significant challenges in self-forgiveness is overcoming the deep-seated guilt and shame that may have been ingrained in you, especially if you have grown up in a toxic family environment where blame and criticism were prevalent. These negative emotions can create a cycle of self-punishment that hinders your ability to heal and grow. This week, we will explore strategies to break this cycle, helping you to let go of these harmful emotions and replace them with self-compassion and understanding.

Self-forgiveness also involves recognizing the difference between healthy accountability and destructive self-blame. Holding yourself accountable for your actions is essential for personal growth, but it should not devolve into relentless self-criticism. We will learn how to strike a balance between acknowledging responsibility and extending compassion to ourselves, fostering a healthier mindset that encourages growth rather than stagnation.

Practicing self-forgiveness can lead to numerous benefits, including improved mental health, increased self-esteem, and stronger, more authentic relationships with others. By releasing the grip of past mistakes, you create space for positive change and self-improvement. This week, we will engage in various exercises and reflections designed to help you embrace self-forgiveness and integrate it into your daily life.

Self-forgiveness is a continuous process that requires patience and practice. It is not a one-time event but an ongoing commitment to treating yourself with the kindness and respect you deserve. As we embark on this week focused on self-forgiveness, embrace the opportunity to release past burdens and move forward with a lighter heart and a more compassionate spirit.

October 15
- **Affirmation:** "I deserve to forgive myself and move forward."
- **Reflection:** "Self-forgiveness is essential for personal growth and healing."
- **Practical Exercise:** Reflect on a mistake you have been holding onto. Write about why you deserve to forgive yourself and how it can help you move forward.

October 16

- **Affirmation:** "I will be gentle with myself as I work through self-forgiveness."
- **Reflection:** "Gentleness and compassion are vital in the process of self-forgiveness."
- **Practical Exercise:** Practice self-compassion by writing a letter to yourself, acknowledging your mistakes and offering forgiveness and understanding.

October 17

- **Affirmation:** "I can learn from my mistakes and grow stronger."
- **Reflection:** "Mistakes are opportunities for learning and growth."
- **Practical Exercise:** Write about a mistake you have made and the lessons you have learned from it. Reflect on how these lessons have contributed to your personal growth.

October 18

- **Affirmation:** "I will let go of self-blame and embrace self-compassion."
- **Reflection:** "Letting go of self-blame is essential for healing and self-acceptance."
- **Practical Exercise:** Reflect on any self-blame you are holding onto. Write about how you can replace self-blame with self-compassion.

October 19

- **Affirmation:** "I am worthy of self-forgiveness and inner peace."
- **Reflection:** "You deserve to forgive yourself and find peace within."
- **Practical Exercise:** Write a forgiveness affirmation specific to yourself. Repeat it daily and reflect on how it impacts your self-perception and peace of mind.

October 20

- **Affirmation:** "I will acknowledge my progress and be patient with myself."

- **Reflection:** "Acknowledging progress and practicing patience is key to self-forgiveness."
- **Practical Exercise:** Reflect on your progress in self-forgiveness. Write about how patience has played a role in your journey.

October 21

- **Affirmation:** "I will celebrate my growth and forgive my past self."
- **Reflection:** "Celebrating growth reinforces the process of self-forgiveness."
- **Practical Exercise:** Reflect on your personal growth and write a letter to your past self, offering forgiveness and celebrating your achievements.

Week 4: Letting Go of Resentment

Introduction of Week's Theme

Letting go of resentment is a powerful and transformative step toward achieving emotional freedom and inner peace. Resentment can linger in your heart and mind, causing ongoing pain and preventing you from moving forward. This week, we will explore understanding the nature of resentment, recognizing its sources, and exploring practical strategies to release it. By letting go of resentment, you can create space for healing, growth, and a more positive mindset.

Resentment often stems from unresolved hurts and perceived injustices. It can arise from past experiences where you felt wronged, betrayed, or unappreciated. These feelings, if left unchecked, can fester and grow, impacting your mental and emotional well-being. Recognizing the specific incidents and emotions that fuel your resentment is the first step in addressing and releasing it. We will begin by identifying the root causes of your resentment and acknowledging the pain it has caused.

One of the most effective ways to let go of resentment is

through the practice of forgiveness. Forgiveness does not mean condoning the hurtful actions of others or forgetting the pain they caused. Instead, it is a conscious decision to release the hold that these negative emotions have on you. This week, we will explore the process of forgiveness, including self-forgiveness, and how it can free you from the burden of resentment. We will discuss practical exercises and reflections that can help you move toward forgiveness.

Mindfulness and self-compassion are crucial tools in the journey to letting go of resentment. By practicing mindfulness, you can become more aware of your thoughts and feelings, allowing you to observe your resentment without judgment. Self-compassion involves being kind and understanding toward yourself as you navigate the difficult process of letting go. This week, we will integrate mindfulness practices and self-compassion techniques to support your emotional healing and foster a more peaceful mindset.

Another key aspect of releasing resentment is reframing your perspective. Holding onto resentment often keeps you stuck in a victim mentality, where you feel powerless and defined by past hurts. By shifting your perspective and focusing on your growth and resilience, you can reclaim your power and transform your outlook. Try reframing your thoughts and cultivating a mindset of empowerment and positivity.

October 22
- **Affirmation:** "I am ready to release resentment and embrace peace."
- **Reflection:** "Releasing resentment allows you to find peace and move forward."
- **Practical Exercise:** Identify a specific resentment you are holding onto. Write about how letting go of this resentment can improve your emotional well-being.

October 23
- **Affirmation:** "I will practice empathy and

understanding to release resentment."

- **Reflection:** "Empathy and understanding can help you see situations from a new perspective."
- **Practical Exercise:** Reflect on a situation where you feel resentment. Write about the perspective of the other person involved and how empathy can help you release your resentment.

October 24

- **Affirmation:** "I choose to let go of anger and embrace forgiveness."
- **Reflection:** "Letting go of anger frees you to experience more positive emotions."
- **Practical Exercise:** Write about a situation where you are holding onto anger. Reflect on how letting go of this anger can open up space for more positive feelings.

October 25

- **Affirmation:** "I will focus on the present and let go of past hurts."
- **Reflection:** "Focusing on the present helps you release the grip of past hurts."
- **Practical Exercise:** Practice mindfulness by focusing on the present moment. Reflect on how being present helps you let go of past resentments.

October 26

- **Affirmation:** "I will replace negative thoughts with positive affirmations."
- **Reflection:** "Positive affirmations can help shift your mindset and release resentment."
- **Practical Exercise:** Write down negative thoughts related to resentment and replace them with positive affirmations. Repeat these affirmations daily and reflect on their impact.

October 27

- **Affirmation:** "I am grateful for the lessons learned and ready to move forward."
- **Reflection:** "Gratitude helps you focus on the positive aspects of your experiences."

- **Practical Exercise:** Write a gratitude list focusing on the lessons you have learned from past resentments. Reflect on how these lessons have helped you grow.

October 28

- **Affirmation:** "I will seek joy and positivity in my daily life."
- **Reflection:** "Seeking joy and positivity helps you maintain a peaceful mindset."
- **Practical Exercise:** Identify activities that bring you joy and incorporate them into your daily routine. Reflect on how these activities help you let go of resentment.

October 29

- **Affirmation:** "I will nurture positive relationships that support my well-being."
- **Reflection:** "Positive relationships reinforce your journey of letting go and healing."
- **Practical Exercise:** Identify relationships that support your well-being. Plan to nurture these connections and reflect on how they enhance your life.

October 30

- **Affirmation:** "I will practice self-care to support my emotional well-being."
- **Reflection:** "Self-care is crucial for maintaining your emotional health."
- **Practical Exercise:** Create a self-care plan that includes activities that nurture your mind, body, and spirit. Reflect on how self-care supports your journey of forgiveness and letting go.

October 31

- **Affirmation:** "I am at peace with my past and excited for my future."
- **Reflection:** "Finding peace with your past allows you to look forward to the future with excitement."
- **Practical Exercise:** Reflect on your past journey of forgiveness and letting go. Write about how finding peace with your past excites you for your future.

October Conclusion

As we conclude our focus on forgiveness and letting go, take a moment to reflect on the progress you have made in releasing past hurts and embracing a more peaceful and positive mindset. Forgiveness is a powerful tool for healing and growth, allowing you to move forward with greater clarity and freedom. The journey of forgiveness is not a linear path but a continuous process that evolves with time and self-awareness.

This month, we explored the true meaning of forgiveness, recognizing that it is not about condoning the actions that hurt you but about freeing yourself from the hold of past grievances. By understanding the importance of forgiveness, you have opened the door to emotional liberation and personal growth, laying the foundation for a more serene and balanced life.

Through practical strategies and reflective exercises, you have learned how to forgive those who have hurt you. This process required courage and vulnerability, as it meant confronting painful memories and choosing to release the hold they had on you. Each act of forgiveness has brought you closer to emotional well-being and inner peace.

Self-forgiveness has been another critical aspect of this journey. Often, we are our harshest critics, holding onto guilt and self-blame for past mistakes. This month, you have focused on being kinder and more compassionate toward yourself, recognizing that self-forgiveness is essential for personal healing. By embracing self-compassion, you have learned to accept your imperfections and celebrate your efforts to grow and improve.

Letting go of resentment has also been a key theme. Resentment can weigh heavily on your heart and mind, preventing you from fully experiencing joy and contentment. Through various strategies, you have practiced releasing resentment and making space for positive emotions, helping you cultivate a more peaceful and harmonious mindset.

Celebrate your progress, acknowledge your strength, and continue to prioritize forgiveness and letting go. Each step you take in this journey brings you closer to a life filled with peace, love, and fulfillment. Embrace the clarity and freedom that forgiveness offers, and let it guide you toward a brighter and more positive future.

November: Living Your Authentic Life

Living your authentic life involves embracing your true self and expressing your genuine thoughts, feelings, and values. It requires a deep understanding of who you are at your core, free from societal expectations and external pressures. This month, we will explore the essence of authenticity, exploring what it means to live a life that is true to your inner self. Authentic living is not just about honesty with others but also about being honest with yourself and acknowledging your true desires, strengths, and areas for growth.

The journey to authenticity begins with self-discovery. Understanding who you are and what you stand for is the foundation of an authentic life. We will start by examining the concept of self-identity and how it shapes your actions, decisions, and interactions with the world. This involves reflecting on your values, passions, and the unique qualities that make you who you are. By gaining clarity on these aspects, you can begin to align your daily life with your true self.

Identifying and overcoming barriers to authenticity is a crucial step in this journey. Many factors can prevent you from living authentically, such as fear of judgment, past traumas, or ingrained societal norms. We will explore these barriers in depth, helping you recognize the specific obstacles that hinder your authenticity. By bringing these issues to light, you can develop strategies to overcome them, allowing you to live more freely and genuinely.

One key aspect of living authentically is expressing yourself openly and honestly. This means communicating your thoughts and feelings with transparency and courage, even when it feels uncomfortable. We will discuss techniques for effective communication that honor your truth while maintaining respect for others. By practicing authentic communication, you can build deeper and more meaningful relationships based on mutual understanding and trust.

Creating a life that reflects your true self also involves making choices that are aligned with your values and passions. We will explore ways to integrate authenticity into various aspects of your life, including your career, relationships, and personal goals. This might involve making significant changes or simply adjusting your perspective to ensure that your actions are in harmony with your authentic self. Living authentically can lead to greater fulfillment and a sense of purpose.

Week 1: Understanding Authenticity

Introduction of Week's Theme

Authenticity involves recognizing your true self and the importance of living in alignment with your values and beliefs. Embracing your true self means acknowledging your unique qualities and living in a way that is true to your core values and beliefs. It means being honest with yourself and others, not conforming to societal pressures or external expectations that don't align with who you truly are. Living authentically has a profound impact on your well-being and relationships.

Fundamental aspects of authenticity include self-awareness, self-acceptance, and self-expression. Self-awareness involves understanding your thoughts, emotions, and behaviors and recognizing how they influence your actions and decisions. Self-acceptance is about embracing your strengths and weaknesses and acknowledging that you are worthy just as you are. Self-expression is the ability to communicate your true self through your actions, words, and choices.

Barriers to authenticity, such as fear of judgment, societal expectations, and internalized beliefs, may prevent you from being your true self. Recognizing these barriers is crucial for overcoming them and moving toward a more authentic way of living. Identifying and challenging these obstacles empowers you to break free from constraints that hinder your authenticity.

Engage in practical exercises designed to enhance your self-awareness and promote authenticity. Reflect on your values, beliefs, and personal experiences to gain a deeper understanding of who you are and what is truly important to you. Trust your inner voice and make decisions that align with your authentic self.

Cultivating relationships that support and respect your true self is also vital. Surround yourself with people who encourage your authenticity and provide a safe space for you to be yourself. Building and maintaining these supportive relationships can significantly enhance your sense of belonging and fulfillment.

By embracing your true self and living in alignment with your values, you can achieve greater self-confidence, improved mental health, and a more fulfilling and meaningful life. Let's embark on this journey together, embracing the power of authenticity to transform your life for the better.

November 1
- **Affirmation:** "I am committed to discovering and embracing my true self."
- **Reflection:** "Understanding your true self is the first step toward living authentically."
- **Practical Exercise:** Reflect on what authenticity means to you. Write about your core values and beliefs and how they define your true self.

November 2

- **Affirmation:** "I will listen to my inner voice and trust my intuition."
- **Reflection:** "Your inner voice and intuition guide you toward authenticity."
- **Practical Exercise:** Spend time in quiet reflection or meditation, focusing on your inner voice. Write about the insights you gain and how they align with your true self.

November 3

- **Affirmation:** "I am worthy of living a life that reflects my true self."
- **Reflection:** "You deserve to live a life that is true to who you are."
- **Practical Exercise:** Write about any doubts or fears you have about living authentically. Reflect on why you are worthy of embracing your true self.

November 4

- **Affirmation:** "I will be honest with myself and others about who I am."
- **Reflection:** "Honesty is a key component of authenticity."
- **Practical Exercise:** Identify an area of your life where you feel you are not being completely honest with yourself or others. Write about how you can start being more truthful in this area.

November 5

- **Affirmation:** "I will celebrate my uniqueness and embrace my individuality."
- **Reflection:** "Your uniqueness is what makes you special. Embrace it."
- **Practical Exercise:** List the unique qualities and traits that make you who you are. Reflect on how these qualities contribute to your authenticity.

November 6

- **Affirmation:** "I will seek clarity about my true desires

and aspirations."
- **Reflection:** "Clarity about your desires helps you live authentically."
- **Practical Exercise:** Spend time journaling about your deepest desires and aspirations. Reflect on how pursuing them aligns with your true self.

November 7
- **Affirmation:** "I am on a journey of self-discovery and growth."
- **Reflection:** "Self-discovery is a continuous process that enriches your life."
- **Practical Exercise:** Reflect on the new aspects of yourself you have discovered recently. Write about how these discoveries contribute to your journey of authenticity.

Week 2: Overcoming Barriers to Authenticity

Introduction of Week's Theme

Living authentically often requires overcoming a range of barriers that can inhibit our true self-expression. This week, we will explore understanding and addressing these barriers, such as fear, societal expectations, and self-doubt, which can significantly impact our ability to live genuinely and wholeheartedly. By identifying these obstacles and developing effective strategies to navigate them, you can move closer to a life that truly reflects who you are at your core.

Fear is one of the most significant barriers to authenticity. Fear of rejection, judgment, or failure can keep you from expressing your true self. It is essential to recognize and confront these fears head-on, understanding that they are a natural part of the human experience. This week, we will explore techniques to manage and reduce fear, allowing you to take bold steps toward authenticity with courage and confidence.

Societal expectations can also impose considerable pressure, often dictating how we should behave, think, or feel. These expectations can come from cultural norms, family traditions, or peer influences, creating an external standard that might not align with your true self. We will examine ways to critically assess these societal pressures, distinguish between external expectations and your personal values, and find the strength to prioritize your own needs and desires.

Self-doubt is another common barrier that can undermine your efforts to live authentically. Doubting your abilities, worth, or decisions can lead to hesitation and second-guessing, preventing you from fully embracing your true self. This week, we will focus on building self-confidence and self-compassion, essential components for overcoming self-doubt. By fostering a positive self-image and trusting in your inherent worth, you can empower yourself to make choices that reflect your genuine self.

Negative past experiences, such as criticism or failure, can leave lasting imprints that fuel fear, societal conformity, and self-doubt. By reflecting on and reinterpreting these experiences, you can begin to dismantle their power over your present life. This process involves acknowledging past wounds, learning from them, and releasing their hold on your identity.

Living authentically is a continuous journey that requires ongoing effort and self-awareness. As you work through the barriers to authenticity, remember that each step forward is a victory. Celebrate your progress, no matter how small, and stay committed to your path. By the end of this week, you will be better equipped to face your fears, challenge societal expectations, and silence self-doubt, paving the way for a life that is true to you.

November 8
- **Affirmation:** "I will face my fears and take steps toward living authentically."
- **Reflection:** "Facing your fears is essential for

embracing your true self."
- **Practical Exercise:** Identify a fear that is holding you back from living authentically. Write about how you can confront and overcome this fear.

November 9
- **Affirmation:** "I will not let societal expectations dictate my life."
- **Reflection:** "Living authentically means being true to yourself, not conforming to others' expectations."
- **Practical Exercise:** Reflect on societal expectations that influence your decisions. Write about how you can resist these pressures and make choices that align with your true self.

November 10
- **Affirmation:** "I am confident in my ability to live authentically."
- **Reflection:** "Confidence in yourself is key to embracing authenticity."
- **Practical Exercise:** Write about a time when you felt truly confident and authentic. Reflect on how you can bring that confidence into other areas of your life.

November 11
- **Affirmation:** "I will challenge and overcome my self-doubt."
- **Reflection:** "Challenging self-doubt is crucial for living an authentic life."
- **Practical Exercise:** Identify areas where self-doubt holds you back. Write affirmations that counter these doubts and reflect on how you can build your self-confidence.

November 12
- **Affirmation:** "I will surround myself with supportive and understanding people."
- **Reflection:** "Supportive relationships encourage and reinforce your authenticity."
- **Practical Exercise:** Reflect on the people in your life who support your true self. Plan to spend more time

with these individuals and seek their encouragement.

November 13
- **Affirmation:** "I will release the need for external validation."
- **Reflection:** "Your authenticity comes from within, not from external approval."
- **Practical Exercise:** Write about times you have sought external validation. Reflect on how you can shift your focus to internal validation and self-acceptance.

November 14
- **Affirmation:** "I am resilient and capable of overcoming obstacles to my authenticity."
- **Reflection:** "Resilience is key to maintaining authenticity in the face of challenges."
- **Practical Exercise:** Identify obstacles you have overcome in the past. Reflect on how these experiences have strengthened your commitment to living authentically.

Week 3: Aligning Your Life with Your True Self

Introduction of Week's Theme

Aligning your life with your true self is a transformative process that requires deep self-reflection and intentional action. It involves recognizing and honoring your core values, passions, and beliefs and ensuring that your daily decisions and actions are congruent with these fundamental aspects of who you are. This week, we will explore the practical steps necessary to achieve this alignment, fostering a life that resonates with your authentic self.

To begin, it's essential to cultivate a clear understanding of your true self. This involves introspection and honest assessment of what truly matters to you. Reflect on your values—those principles that guide your decisions and actions. Consider your passions, the activities and interests that bring you joy and fulfillment. Acknowledge your beliefs and the convictions that shape your worldview and influence your behavior. By gaining clarity on these aspects, you lay the foundation for living a life aligned with your true self.

Once you have a clear understanding of your true self, the next step is to evaluate your current life circumstances. Examine how your daily routines, relationships, and professional pursuits align with your core values, passions, and beliefs. Identify any areas of misalignment where your actions and choices do not reflect your authentic self. This evaluation process is crucial for pinpointing the changes needed to bring your life into alignment with your true self.

Making changes to align your life with your true self often involves setting new priorities and goals. Establish clear, actionable steps to adjust your lifestyle, focusing on areas that require realignment. This might mean pursuing a career that aligns with your passions, fostering relationships that support your values, or incorporating daily practices that nurture your beliefs. Setting specific, measurable goals will help you track your progress and stay committed to the journey of alignment.

As you begin to make these changes, it's important to practice self-compassion and patience. Aligning your life with your true self is a continuous journey that involves trial and error. There may be setbacks and challenges along the way, but each step forward is a testament to your commitment to living authentically. Celebrate your progress, no matter how small, and remind yourself that every effort counts toward creating a life that reflects your true self.

Seeking support from others can also play a significant role in this process. Surround yourself with individuals who understand and respect your journey toward authenticity. Share your goals and challenges with trusted friends, family members, or mentors who can offer encouragement and guidance. Consider joining groups or communities that share your values and interests, providing a sense of belonging and reinforcement as you align your life with your true self.

Finally, remember that aligning your life with your true self is an ongoing process that evolves as you grow and change. Regularly revisit your values, passions, and beliefs, and adjust your actions and goals accordingly. Stay open to new experiences and insights that can further enhance your understanding of your true self. By continually aligning your life with your authenticity, you pave the way for a fulfilling and meaningful existence that resonates deeply with who you are.

November 15
- **Affirmation:** "I will make choices that reflect my values and beliefs."
- **Reflection:** "Your choices should align with what is important to you."
- **Practical Exercise:** Identify an area of your life where your actions do not fully align with your values. Write about the changes you can make to bring this area into alignment.

November 16
- **Affirmation:** "I will pursue my passions and interests with enthusiasm."
- **Reflection:** "Pursuing your passions is a key aspect of living authentically."
- **Practical Exercise:** Write about your passions and interests. Make a plan to dedicate time to these pursuits and reflect on how they contribute to your authenticity.

November 17
- **Affirmation:** "I will set goals that align with my true self."
- **Reflection:** "Goals that reflect your true self lead to a more fulfilling life."
- **Practical Exercise:** Set short-term and long-term goals that align with your values and passions. Reflect on the steps you need to take to achieve these goals.

November 18

- **Affirmation:** "I will practice self-care to support my authentic self."
- **Reflection:** "Self-care is essential for maintaining your authenticity."
- **Practical Exercise:** Create a self-care plan that nurtures your mind, body, and spirit. Reflect on how self-care supports your journey toward authenticity.

November 19

- **Affirmation:** "I will take risks and embrace new opportunities for growth."
- **Reflection:** "Taking risks can lead to personal growth and greater authenticity."
- **Practical Exercise:** Identify a risk or new opportunity that aligns with your true self. Make a plan to take this risk and reflect on how it can help you grow.

November 20

- **Affirmation:** "I will seek balance in my life to support my authenticity."
- **Reflection:** "Balance in life supports your ability to live authentically."
- **Practical Exercise:** Reflect on areas where you may need more balance. Write about how achieving balance in these areas can support your authenticity.

November 21

- **Affirmation:** "I will nurture relationships that honor my true self."
- **Reflection:** "Relationships that honor your true self support your authenticity."
- **Practical Exercise:** Identify relationships that support your authenticity. Plan ways to nurture these relationships and reflect on their positive impact on your life.

Week 4: Embracing and Celebrating Your Authentic Life

Introduction of Week's Theme

Embracing and celebrating your authentic life is a multifaceted journey that involves recognizing your achievements, expressing gratitude, and continuously striving to live in alignment with your true self. This week, we will explore the importance of acknowledging your progress, understanding the power of gratitude, and setting intentions that honor your authentic path. Living authentically means embracing who you truly are, free from the constraints of societal expectations or toxic influences. This week is dedicated to celebrating that freedom and reinforcing your commitment to your personal growth.

One key aspect of embracing your authentic life is recognizing your achievements. Throughout your journey, you have faced numerous challenges and made significant strides in your personal development. Taking the time to reflect on these accomplishments is crucial. This recognition not only boosts your self-esteem but also reinforces the positive changes you have made. It is an affirmation of your resilience and a reminder of your capability to overcome obstacles. Celebrating your achievements, no matter how small, is a vital step in nurturing your authentic self.

Expressing gratitude is another powerful tool for embracing your authentic life. Gratitude shifts your focus from what is lacking to what is abundant. It helps you appreciate the present moment and the progress you have made. This week, we will explore various gratitude practices that can enhance your well-being and foster a positive mindset. By regularly acknowledging the positive aspects of your life, you create a foundation of contentment and joy, which supports your journey toward authenticity.

Living in alignment with your true self requires continuous effort and intentionality. It involves making choices that reflect your values, passions, and aspirations. This week, we will focus on setting intentions that guide you toward a fulfilling and authentic life. Intentions are powerful because they provide direction and purpose. They help you stay committed to your path and navigate through life's challenges with clarity and confidence. By setting clear and meaningful intentions, you can create a roadmap for your journey toward a more authentic life.

Self-expression is a critical component of living authentically. It involves sharing your true thoughts, feelings, and desires without fear of judgment or rejection. This week, we will explore ways to enhance your self-expression and communicate your authenticity to the world. Whether through creative outlets, honest conversations, or personal projects, expressing yourself fully allows you to live more genuinely. It also strengthens your relationships, as others are drawn to your authenticity and honesty.

November 22
- **Affirmation:** "I will celebrate my journey toward authenticity."
- **Reflection:** "Celebrating your progress reinforces your commitment to authenticity."
- **Practical Exercise:** Reflect on your journey toward living authentically. Write about your achievements and how they have positively impacted your life.

November 23
- **Affirmation:** "I will express gratitude for my authentic self."
- **Reflection:** "Gratitude for your true self fosters self-acceptance and joy."
- **Practical Exercise:** Write a gratitude list focusing on the aspects of your true self that you appreciate. Reflect on how gratitude enhances your self-perception.

November 24
- **Affirmation:** "I will continue to grow and evolve in my authenticity."

- **Reflection:** "Personal growth is a continuous journey that enhances your authenticity."
- **Practical Exercise:** Identify areas where you want to continue growing. Write about the steps you will take to foster this growth and embrace your evolving self.

November 25
- **Affirmation:** "I will inspire others by living authentically."
- **Reflection:** "Living authentically can inspire and encourage others to do the same."
- **Practical Exercise:** Reflect on how your journey toward authenticity can inspire others. Write about ways you can share your experiences and encourage others to embrace their true selves.

November 26
- **Affirmation:** "I am proud of who I am and the life I am creating."
- **Reflection:** "Pride in your authentic self reinforces your commitment to living truthfully."
- **Practical Exercise:** Write a letter to yourself expressing pride in your journey and the life you are creating. Reflect on how this pride motivates you to continue living authentically.

November 27
- **Affirmation:** "I will maintain balance in my life to support my authenticity."
- **Reflection:** "Balance in life supports your ability to live authentically."
- **Practical Exercise:** Reflect on areas where you may need more balance. Write about how achieving balance in these areas can support your authenticity.

November 28
- **Affirmation:** "I will seek joy and fulfillment in living my authentic life."
- **Reflection:** "Joy and fulfillment are the rewards of living authentically."
- **Practical Exercise:** Identify activities and

relationships that bring you joy and fulfillment. Make a plan to incorporate more of these elements into your life.

November 29
- **Affirmation:** "I will forgive myself for any past compromises of my authenticity."
- **Reflection:** "Self-forgiveness is important for moving forward with authenticity."
- **Practical Exercise:** Write about any past compromises of your authenticity. Reflect on how forgiving yourself can free you to live more truthfully now.

November 30
- **Affirmation:** "I am committed to living my life authentically and fully."
- **Reflection:** "Commitment to authenticity enriches your life and relationships."
- **Practical Exercise:** Write a declaration of commitment to living authentically. Reflect on how this commitment will guide your actions and decisions moving forward.

November Conclusion

Reflect on the significant progress made in understanding, embracing, and expressing your true self throughout this month focused on living authentically. Living authentically is not a destination but a continuous journey requiring ongoing self-awareness, courage, and dedication.

This month, you identified and began addressing barriers preventing you from living authentically. These barriers, whether internal fears, societal expectations, or self-doubt, often seem insurmountable. However, recognizing and confronting them has started the process of dismantling these obstacles, paving the way for a life true to who you are.

Aligning your life with your core values and passions is

a crucial step in living authentically. This alignment allows for choices consistent with your true self, leading to greater satisfaction and happiness. Practical steps to integrate your values into daily life have moved you closer to a life that brings joy and fulfillment. This commitment to living genuinely is commendable and demonstrates dedication to personal growth.

Embracing your authenticity also involves celebrating your unique journey and the progress made. Each step, no matter how small, is a victory worth acknowledging. Setting intentions for continued growth ensures that you remain on the path to authenticity, navigating life's complexities while staying true to yourself. Celebrate your achievements and use them as motivation to keep moving forward.

Reflect on the skills acquired this month: a deeper understanding of what it means to be authentic and the numerous benefits it brings, strategies to overcome barriers, and practical steps to align your life with your true self. Embracing authenticity has set the stage for continued growth and self-discovery.

Celebrate your progress, acknowledge your strength, and continue to prioritize authenticity in all aspects of your life. The journey toward living authentically is ongoing, and each step brings you closer to a life that is truly your own. Move forward with confidence and self-compassion, knowing that you are building a future that reflects your true self.

December: Continuing the Healing Journey

The journey of healing is ongoing, and each step forward brings you closer to a more fulfilled and balanced life. This month, we will focus on strategies to sustain your progress, embrace continuous growth, and prepare for the future with hope and resilience. By reflecting on your journey, setting new goals, and nurturing your well-being, you can maintain the momentum of your healing process and continue to thrive. Let's dedicate this month to reinforcing the positive changes you've made and envisioning a bright and fulfilling future.

Healing is not a destination but a continuous journey that evolves as you grow and change. It is essential to recognize the progress you have made while understanding that there is always room for further growth. This month, we will take time to reflect on the strides you have made throughout the year. Acknowledging your achievements, no matter how small, is crucial for reinforcing positive changes and building confidence in your ability to continue healing.

One key aspect of maintaining your healing journey is setting new, achievable goals. These goals should align with your values and aspirations, providing a clear direction for your continued growth. We will explore realistic and motivating goal-setting techniques, helping you stay focused and committed to your path. By setting these goals, you create a roadmap for your ongoing journey, ensuring that you remain proactive in your healing process.

Self-care remains a cornerstone of your healing journey. This month, we will explore advanced self-care practices that nurture your body, mind and spirit. These practices include mindfulness techniques, creative expression, and physical activities that promote overall well-being. By prioritizing self-care, you ensure that you have the energy and resilience to face any challenges that come your way.

Reflecting on your support system is another crucial element of sustaining your healing journey. We will examine the relationships and resources that have supported you thus far and consider ways to strengthen these connections. Whether it's friends, family, or professional support, maintaining a robust support network is vital for ongoing healing. We will also explore ways to expand your support system, ensuring you have the help and encouragement you need.

Embracing continuous growth involves staying open to new experiences and learning opportunities. This month, we will focus on cultivating a growth mindset, which encourages you to see challenges as opportunities for development rather than obstacles. By fostering a mindset of continuous improvement, you remain adaptable and resilient, ready to navigate whatever comes your way.

Week 1: Reflecting on Your Progress

Introduction of Week's Theme

Reflecting on your progress is a crucial aspect of personal growth and self-awareness. This week, we will explore the practice of self-reflection, which allows you to recognize and celebrate how far you've come while also identifying areas that may still need attention and improvement. Taking the time to reflect on your journey can provide valuable insights and motivation, reinforcing your commitment to ongoing growth and healing.

Self-reflection serves as a powerful tool for acknowledging your achievements and the positive changes you've made in your life. By looking back on your experiences and accomplishments, you can see the tangible results of your efforts. This recognition not only boosts your confidence but also encourages you to continue striving toward your goals. Each milestone, no matter how small, is a testament to your resilience and determination.

Throughout this week, we will explore various methods and techniques for effective self-reflection. These methods may include journaling, meditation, and discussions with trusted friends or mentors. Journaling, in particular, provides a written record of your thoughts and experiences, allowing you to track your progress over time. Meditation can help you gain clarity and focus, making it easier to assess your journey objectively. Conversations with others can offer new perspectives and reinforce the positive changes you've made.

We will also focus on the importance of celebrating your successes. Acknowledging your progress isn't just about identifying areas for improvement; it's about giving yourself credit for the hard work you've put in. Celebrations can take many forms, from treating yourself to something special to simply taking a moment to appreciate your achievements. By celebrating your successes, you reinforce the positive behaviors and habits that have contributed to your growth.

Another key aspect of reflecting on your progress is identifying the strategies and actions that have been most effective for you. By understanding what has worked well, you can continue to apply these strategies in the future. Additionally, recognizing any setbacks or challenges you've faced can help you develop better-coping mechanisms and adjust your approach moving forward. Reflection is not just about looking back; it's about learning and growing from your experiences.

As we progress through this week, remember that self-reflection is an ongoing process. It's something you can integrate into your daily routine to monitor your progress and make necessary adjustments continually. This practice will help you stay aligned with your goals and maintain a sense of purpose and direction. Embrace this opportunity to reflect on your journey, celebrate your achievements, and set the stage for future growth.

Ultimately, reflecting on your progress is about honoring your journey and recognizing the strength and resilience that have brought you this far. It's a chance to appreciate the person you've become and to feel proud of your accomplishments. By dedicating this week to reflection, you are taking an important step in your ongoing journey of self-discovery and personal growth.

December 1

- **Affirmation:** "I am proud of the progress I have made on my healing journey."
- **Reflection:** "Acknowledging your progress reinforces your commitment to healing."
- **Practical Exercise:** Write about the significant milestones you've achieved this year. Reflect on how these accomplishments have impacted your life positively.

December 2

- **Affirmation:** "I will celebrate my successes, no matter how small."
- **Reflection:** "Every success is a step forward on your journey."
- **Practical Exercise:** List small victories you've experienced recently. Reflect on how celebrating these successes boosts your confidence and motivation.

December 3

- **Affirmation:** "I will acknowledge the challenges I have overcome."
- **Reflection:** "Recognizing the challenges you've faced shows your resilience."
- **Practical Exercise:** Reflect on a challenging situation you overcame this year. Write about the strengths and skills you used to navigate it.

December 4

- **Affirmation:** "I am grateful for the lessons I have learned on my journey."
- **Reflection:** "Gratitude for your experiences enhances your growth."
- **Practical Exercise:** Write a gratitude list focusing on the lessons you've learned. Reflect on how these lessons have contributed to your personal growth.

December 5

- **Affirmation:** "I will continue to reflect on my journey to understand my growth."
- **Reflection:** "Continuous reflection helps you stay aware of your progress."
- **Practical Exercise:** Spend time journaling about your healing journey. Reflect on how self-reflection has helped you understand and appreciate your growth.

December 6

- **Affirmation:** "I will use my past experiences as a foundation for future growth."
- **Reflection:** "Your past experiences shape your present and future."
- **Practical Exercise:** Write about how your past experiences have prepared you for future challenges and opportunities.

December 7

- **Affirmation:** "I am committed to ongoing self-improvement and personal growth."
- **Reflection:** "Commitment to growth is key to a fulfilling life."
- **Practical Exercise:** Set an intention for continuous

self-improvement. Write about the steps you will take to achieve this.

Week 2: Setting New Goals for Growth

Introduction of Week's Theme

Setting new goals is an essential part of maintaining momentum and ensuring continuous personal growth. Goals provide direction, motivation, and a sense of purpose, helping you to keep moving forward in your journey. This week, we will explore the importance of setting new aspirations, how to identify them, and the steps needed to create actionable plans to achieve them. By the end of this week, you will have a clear roadmap to guide you toward your next milestones.

First, we will explore the significance of goal-setting in personal development. Goals are not just targets to hit; they represent your desires, ambitions, and the steps you take to reach your full potential. Setting new goals keeps you engaged and prevents stagnation, ensuring that you are always moving toward something meaningful. We will discuss how setting specific, measurable, achievable, relevant, and time-bound (SMART) goals can provide a structured approach to achieving your aspirations.

Identifying new aspirations begins with self-reflection. This involves taking a step back to assess where you are currently and where you want to go. Reflect on your achievements so far and consider areas where you feel there is room for growth. We will guide you through exercises to help you uncover your true passions and interests, which can then be transformed into concrete goals. This process of self-discovery is crucial for setting goals that resonate deeply with you.

Once you have identified your aspirations, the next step is to break them down into actionable plans. This involves setting smaller, manageable steps that will lead you toward your larger objectives. We will discuss how to prioritize these steps, allocate resources, and create timelines to keep you on track. By breaking down your goals into bite-sized tasks, you make the journey more manageable and less overwhelming, increasing your chances of success.

We will also address the potential obstacles that might arise as you pursue your goals. It is important to anticipate challenges and prepare strategies to overcome them. This includes building resilience, seeking support, and staying flexible. We will provide tips on how to stay motivated, handle setbacks, and maintain a positive mindset throughout your journey. Remember, the path to achieving your goals is rarely linear, and being prepared for bumps along the way will help you stay focused.

Throughout this week, you will engage in practical exercises designed to solidify your goals and plans. These exercises will help you visualize your future, create detailed action plans, and set milestones to track your progress. By the end of the week, you will have a comprehensive plan that outlines your goals, the steps to achieve them, and the strategies to handle challenges. This plan will serve as a roadmap, guiding you toward continuous growth and personal development.

In summary, setting new goals is a dynamic and ongoing process that fuels your personal growth. This week is dedicated to helping you identify your aspirations, create actionable plans, and develop the resilience needed to achieve your dreams. Embrace this opportunity to focus on your future, set meaningful goals, and take decisive steps toward realizing your full potential. Let's embark on this journey together, with confidence and determination, to create the life you envision.

December 8
  - **Affirmation:** "I will set goals that align with my values and aspirations."
  - **Reflection:** "Goals that reflect your values lead to a

more fulfilling life."
- **Practical Exercise:** Reflect on your core values and aspirations. Write down new goals that align with these principles and detail the steps needed to achieve them.

December 9
- **Affirmation:** "I will break down my goals into manageable steps."
- **Reflection:** "Breaking down goals makes them more achievable."
- **Practical Exercise:** Take one of your new goals and break it down into smaller, manageable tasks. Create a timeline for completing each step.

December 10
- **Affirmation:** "I will stay committed to my personal growth and development."
- **Reflection:** "Commitment to growth ensures continuous progress."
- **Practical Exercise:** Write a commitment statement to yourself about staying dedicated to your personal growth. Reflect on how this commitment will guide your actions.

December 11
- **Affirmation:** "I will embrace challenges as opportunities for growth."
- **Reflection:** "Challenges can be powerful catalysts for growth."
- **Practical Exercise:** Reflect on a recent challenge and write about how it can be an opportunity for personal development. Plan how you will approach similar challenges in the future.

December 12
- **Affirmation:** "I will celebrate my progress and set new milestones."
- **Reflection:** "Celebrating progress motivates you to continue setting new goals."
- **Practical Exercise:** Identify a recent achievement and

celebrate it in a meaningful way. Set a new milestone that builds on this achievement.

December 13
- **Affirmation:** "I will stay flexible and adapt to new circumstances."
- **Reflection:** "Flexibility helps you navigate changes and continue growing."
- **Practical Exercise:** Reflect on a recent change or challenge. Write about how staying flexible helped you adapt and what you learned from the experience.

December 14
- **Affirmation:** "I will set clear intentions for the coming year."
- **Reflection:** "Setting intentions helps you stay focused and motivated."
- **Practical Exercise:** Write down your intentions for the coming year. Reflect on how these intentions align with your values and goals.

Week 3: Nurturing Your Well-Being

Introduction of Week's Theme

Nurturing your well-being is essential for sustaining your progress and maintaining a healthy, balanced life. This week, we will explore various strategies and practices to prioritize self-care and ensure your physical, emotional, and mental well-being. By committing to these practices, you can build resilience, improve your overall health, and create a more fulfilling life.

Self-care is more than just occasional pampering; it is a consistent and intentional practice of taking care of your mind, body, and spirit. This involves recognizing and addressing your needs, setting boundaries, and making time for activities that rejuvenate and energize you. Throughout this week, we will explore different aspects of self-care, from physical activities and nutrition to emotional support and mental clarity.

Physical well-being is a foundational aspect of self-care. It encompasses regular exercise, balanced nutrition, adequate sleep, and routine medical check-ups. Engaging in physical activities you enjoy, such as walking, yoga, or dancing, can boost your mood and energy levels. Similarly, nourishing your body with healthy foods and staying hydrated are crucial for maintaining your health and vitality. This week, we will discuss practical tips and exercises to help you incorporate physical self-care into your daily routine.

Emotional well-being involves understanding and managing your emotions effectively. This includes acknowledging your feelings, expressing them in healthy ways, and seeking support when needed. Building a strong support system of friends, family, or professionals can provide the emotional nourishment you need. We will explore techniques for emotional regulation, such as journaling, mindfulness, and therapy, which can help you navigate your emotions and maintain emotional balance.

Mental well-being is about cultivating a positive mindset and maintaining mental clarity. This can be achieved through practices such as mindfulness, meditation, and positive affirmations. Engaging in activities that stimulate your mind, such as reading, puzzles, or learning new skills, can also contribute to your mental health. This week, we will examine ways to challenge negative thoughts, reduce stress, and promote mental clarity through various cognitive and mindfulness exercises.

Spiritual well-being, though often overlooked, is an important aspect of overall health. It involves finding meaning and purpose in life, connecting with something greater than yourself, and nurturing your inner self. This can be achieved through practices such as meditation, prayer, spending time in nature, or engaging in activities that align with your values and passions. We will explore different ways to nurture your spiritual well-being and create a sense of inner peace and fulfillment.

By the end of this week, you will have a comprehensive toolkit of self-care strategies to nurture your well-being across all aspects of your life. Remember, self-care is not a luxury but a necessity for maintaining your health and happiness. Embrace these practices with commitment and compassion, knowing that taking care of yourself is the first step toward leading a balanced and fulfilling life.

December 15
- **Affirmation:** "I will prioritize self-care to maintain my well-being."
- **Reflection:** "Self-care is essential for overall health and happiness."
- **Practical Exercise:** Create a self-care plan that includes activities for your mind, body, and spirit. Commit to practicing one self-care activity daily.

December 16
- **Affirmation:** "I will listen to my body and respond to its needs."
- **Reflection:** "Listening to your body helps you stay attuned to your health."
- **Practical Exercise:** Practice a body scan meditation to check in with your physical state. Reflect on any areas of tension or discomfort and how you can address them.

December 17
- **Affirmation:** "I will practice mindfulness to stay present and reduce stress."
- **Reflection:** "Mindfulness helps you stay grounded and focused."
- **Practical Exercise:** Spend time practicing mindfulness meditation or mindful breathing. Reflect on how staying present reduces stress and enhances your well-being.

December 18

- **Affirmation:** "I will seek support when needed to nurture my well-being."
- **Reflection:** "Seeking support is a sign of strength and self-awareness."
- **Practical Exercise:** Identify support systems available to you (e.g., friends, family, professionals). Make a plan to reach out for support when you need it.

December 19

- **Affirmation:** "I will maintain a balanced lifestyle to support my growth."
- **Reflection:** "Balance in life is key to sustaining progress and well-being."
- **Practical Exercise:** Reflect on areas where you may need more balance (e.g., work, relationships, leisure). Write about steps you can take to create a more balanced lifestyle.

December 20

- **Affirmation:** "I will nurture my passions and hobbies."
- **Reflection:** "Pursuing your passions enriches your life and brings joy."
- **Practical Exercise:** Write about your passions and hobbies. Plan to dedicate time to these activities regularly and reflect on how they enhance your well-being.

December 21

- **Affirmation:** "I will practice gratitude for the progress I have made."
- **Reflection:** "Gratitude reinforces your commitment to growth and healing."
- **Practical Exercise:** Write a gratitude list focusing on the progress you've made this year. Reflect on how gratitude enhances your perspective and motivation.

Week 4: Preparing for the Future

Introduction of Week's Theme

Preparing for the future with hope and resilience is essential for continued growth and thriving. This week, we will focus on envisioning your future, setting intentions, cultivating a positive outlook, and building on the progress you've made in identifying and transforming toxic thinking patterns.

Envisioning your future is a powerful exercise that allows you to create a mental image of the life you want to lead. This visualization process helps clarify your goals and aspirations, making them more tangible and achievable. We will guide you through techniques to create a vivid and inspiring vision for your future, emphasizing the importance of aligning this vision with your core values and desires.

Setting intentions is a crucial step in turning your vision into reality. Intentions are the guiding principles that shape your actions and decisions, ensuring that you stay focused on your goals. This week, we will explore how to set clear, actionable intentions that reflect your aspirations and support your journey toward a healthier, more fulfilling life. By setting intentions, you create a roadmap that directs your energy and efforts toward achieving your dreams.

Cultivating a positive outlook is vital for maintaining hope and resilience. A positive mindset enables you to approach challenges with confidence and optimism, viewing setbacks as opportunities for growth rather than obstacles. We will explore strategies for fostering a positive outlook, including gratitude practices, positive affirmations, and mindfulness techniques. These practices will help you stay grounded in the present while maintaining a hopeful perspective on the future.

December 22

- **Affirmation:** "I will envision a positive and fulfilling future."
- **Reflection:** "A positive vision for the future motivates and inspires you."
- **Practical Exercise:** Spend time visualizing your ideal

future. Write about what it looks like and how you feel about living that life.

December 23
- **Affirmation:** "I will cultivate a mindset of abundance and possibility."
- **Reflection:** "An abundance mindset helps you see opportunities and potential."
- **Practical Exercise:** Reflect on areas where you may have a scarcity mindset. Write about how you can shift to an abundance mindset and embrace possibilities.

December 24
- **Affirmation:** "I will build strong and supportive relationships."
- **Reflection:** "Supportive relationships are crucial for your well-being."
- **Practical Exercise:** Reflect on the relationships in your life. Write about how you can strengthen these connections and seek new supportive relationships.

December 25
- **Affirmation:** "I will maintain a healthy work-life balance."
- **Reflection:** "A healthy balance between work and personal life supports overall well-being."
- **Practical Exercise:** Reflect on your current work-life balance. Write about steps you can take to improve this balance in the coming year.

December 26
- **Affirmation:** "I will stay resilient in the face of challenges."
- **Reflection:** "Resilience helps you navigate obstacles and continue growing."
- **Practical Exercise:** Reflect on a time when you demonstrated resilience. Write about the strategies you used and how you can apply them to future challenges.

December 27

- **Affirmation:** "I will seek joy and fulfillment in everyday moments."
- **Reflection:** "Finding joy in daily life enhances your overall happiness."
- **Practical Exercise:** Identify simple activities that bring you joy. Make a plan to incorporate these activities into your daily routine and reflect on their impact.

December 28

- **Affirmation:** "I will continue to invest in my well-being and happiness."
- **Reflection:** "Investing in your well-being ensures a fulfilling life."
- **Practical Exercise:** Reflect on the ways you invest in your well-being. Write about new strategies you can implement to enhance your happiness and health.

December 29

- **Affirmation:** "I will stay committed to my personal and professional growth."
- **Reflection:** "Commitment to growth ensures continuous improvement."
- **Practical Exercise:** Set personal and professional growth goals for the coming year. Reflect on the actions needed to achieve these goals.

December 30

- **Affirmation:** "I will honor my journey and celebrate my growth."
- **Reflection:** "Honoring your journey reinforces your commitment to healing."
- **Practical Exercise:** Write about your healing journey and the growth you've experienced. Celebrate your progress in a meaningful way.

December 31

- **Affirmation:** "I am ready to embrace the future with hope and resilience."
- **Reflection:** "Hope and resilience guide you toward a brighter future."
- **Practical Exercise:** Write a letter to your future self,

expressing hope and setting intentions for the coming year. Reflect on the excitement and possibilities that lie ahead.

December Conclusion

As we conclude this month focused on continuing the healing journey, take a moment to reflect on the progress you have made, the goals you have set, and the strategies you have implemented to nurture your well-being. The journey of healing is continuous, and each step forward brings you closer to a more balanced and fulfilling life.

By reflecting on your progress, setting new goals, nurturing your well-being, and preparing for the future, you have reinforced your commitment to personal growth and resilience. Remember, you have the strength and capacity to continue healing and thriving.

Celebrate your journey, acknowledge your efforts, and look forward to the future with hope and confidence. Keep moving forward with self-compassion and determination, knowing that each step you take brings you closer to a life filled with peace, joy, and fulfillment.

Conclusion

As we reach the end of our time together, pause to honor the remarkable journey you have undertaken. This year has been a profound exploration of your past, present, and future, woven with moments of introspection, growth, and transformation. You have bravely explored the complexities of toxic family dynamics, uncovering the deep-seated patterns and behaviors that have shaped your life. This courageous journey has not been easy, but every step you have taken is a testament to your resilience and strength.

Over the past year, you have learned to set boundaries, an essential skill for protecting your well-being and nurturing healthy relationships. You have discovered the vital importance of self-care, understanding that taking care of yourself is not a luxury but a necessity. Through daily affirmations and reflections, you have cultivated self-love, recognizing your inherent worth and beauty. Each month's theme was carefully designed to build upon the previous one, creating a holistic path to healing.

You have explored forgiveness not as a way to excuse the actions of others but as a powerful tool to release yourself from the chains of anger and resentment. Embracing authenticity has allowed you to reclaim your true self, shedding the masks you once wore to protect yourself. You have cultivated a supportive network, understanding that you do not have to walk this path alone. Along the way, you have challenged toxic thoughts, reframing them with positive affirmations and self-compassion, which has been crucial in rebuilding your self-esteem.

Reflecting on this journey, you can see how each theme, each exercise, and each moment of reflection has woven together to create a tapestry of healing and growth. The progress you have made is profound. You have moved from a place of pain and confusion to one of clarity and strength. You have transformed your wounds into wisdom and your struggles into strengths. This journey has been more than just a path to healing; it has been a spiritual awakening, a rediscovery of your true self, and a reclaiming of your life.

Take a moment to acknowledge the depth of your commitment and the courage it took to embark on this journey. Each step forward, no matter how small, has contributed to the beautiful transformation you have undergone. Your dedication to healing is a powerful testament to your resilience, a shining beacon of hope for what lies ahead. As you reflect on your journey, know that you have not only survived but thrived, turning your past into a source of strength and empowerment. You are living proof that healing is possible and that with perseverance and self-compassion, a brighter, more authentic future is within reach.

Reinforce Key Messages
Throughout this book, several key messages have been emphasized repeatedly because they are fundamental to your healing and growth. Each month, we explored specific themes that build on one another, creating a broad framework for overcoming toxic family dynamics and fostering personal development. The journey you have embarked on is filled with powerful lessons and essential practices that can transform your life.

January: Understanding Toxic Families
In January, we focused on understanding the dynamics of toxic families. Recognizing the signs of toxic behavior and acknowledging its impact on your well-being is the first step in

your healing journey. Through daily affirmations, we reinforced the message that you are worthy of a loving and supportive environment. Reflecting on these experiences helped you gain clarity and validate your feelings. By identifying toxic patterns, you set the foundation for change and prepare yourself for the work ahead.

February: Coping with Your Toxic Family
February emphasized coping strategies for dealing with toxic family members. We explored healthy coping mechanisms, such as setting boundaries and practicing self-care, while highlighting the importance of avoiding unhealthy behaviors like substance abuse and excessive people-pleasing. Affirmations and reflections this month focused on resilience and self-protection, empowering you to manage interactions with toxic individuals without compromising your mental health. By applying these strategies, you built a toolkit for navigating difficult family dynamics.

March: When to Cut Ties and Walk Away
In March, we faced the difficult decision of when to cut ties and walk away from toxic relationships. This month's affirmations reinforced your right to prioritize your well-being and make choices that support your mental health. We explored the emotional and practical aspects of ending harmful relationships, including how to recognize the signs that it's time to walk away and the steps to do so safely. Reflecting on these decisions helped you understand that sometimes, the healthiest option is to distance yourself from toxic influences.

April: Boundaries and Healthy Relationships
April was dedicated to the critical practice of setting and maintaining boundaries. This month, we focused on the different types of boundaries—emotional, physical, and mental—and how they protect your well-being. Affirmations encourage you to assert your needs and stand firm in your

limits. Reflections helped you identify areas in your life where boundaries were lacking and develop strategies to enforce them. Building healthy relationships starts with respecting your own boundaries and expecting the same from others.

May: Self-Care and Recovery

May highlighted the importance of self-care and recovery. We explored various self-care practices, such as journaling, meditation, and physical activities, that promote healing and well-being. Affirmations this month reminded you that self-care is not selfish but essential for recovery. Reflecting on your self-care routines helped you identify what truly nurtures you and incorporate these practices into your daily life. By prioritizing self-care, you laid a strong foundation for sustained healing and growth.

June: Getting Help When Needed

In June, we focused on the importance of seeking help when needed. Whether it's through therapy, support groups, or trusted friends, reaching out for support is a sign of strength, not weakness. Affirmations encourage you to embrace vulnerability and ask for help without shame. Reflections helped you identify your support network and understand how to make the most of the resources available to you. By seeking and accepting help, you acknowledge that you don't have to face your challenges alone.

July: Stop Toxic Thinking

July was dedicated to identifying and challenging toxic thought patterns. We explored cognitive distortions, negative core beliefs, and the inner critic that can undermine your self-esteem and mental health. Affirmations focused on cultivating a positive mindset and reframing negative thoughts. Reflections encourage mindfulness and self-awareness, helping you observe your thoughts without judgment and replacing toxic thinking with healthier perspectives. By addressing your thought patterns, you took control of your mental narrative and promoted positive change.

August: Rebuilding Self-Esteem

In August, we worked on rebuilding self-esteem and fostering self-love. This month's affirmations reinforced your inherent worth and encouraged self-compassion. Reflections helped you identify past experiences that damaged your self-esteem and develop strategies to rebuild it. We explored the power of positive self-talk, celebrating your strengths, and acknowledging your achievements. By focusing on self-esteem, you strengthen your foundation for a more confident and authentic life.

September: Creating a Support System

September emphasized the importance of creating a support system. We explored how to identify supportive individuals, build trusting relationships, and maintain a network of people who uplift and encourage you. Affirmations highlighted the value of community and mutual support. Reflections help you assess your current relationships and make intentional efforts to cultivate a strong support system. By surrounding yourself with positive influences, you create a buffer against toxicity and a source of strength.

October: Forgiveness and Letting Go

In October, we explored the challenging process of forgiveness and letting go. Affirmations encourage you to release resentment and embrace the freedom that comes with forgiveness. Reflections helped you understand the difference between forgiving and condoning harmful behavior. We explored practical steps to forgive others and yourself, emphasizing the healing power of letting go. By practicing forgiveness, you freed yourself from the burden of past hurts and made space for peace and growth.

November: Living Your Authentic Life

November focused on embracing and living your authentic life. Affirmations celebrate your unique qualities and encourage you to express your true self. Reflections guided you in identifying areas where you might be compromising your authenticity and how to make changes that align with your values. We explored the importance of pursuing your passions, setting authentic goals, and building a life that reflects who you truly are. By living authentically, you created a life of fulfillment and joy.

December: Continuing the Healing Journey
Finally, in December, we reflected on your progress and set intentions for continued growth. Affirmations reinforced the idea that healing is a continuous journey, not a destination. Reflections helped you celebrate your achievements and recognize the ongoing nature of personal development. We explored strategies to maintain your progress, set new goals, and stay committed to your healing journey. By acknowledging the continuous nature of growth, you embraced a mindset of lifelong learning and resilience.

These key messages—understanding toxic dynamics, setting boundaries, practicing self-care, seeking help, challenging toxic thoughts, rebuilding self-esteem, creating a support system, forgiving and letting go, living authentically, and continuing your healing journey—are the pillars of your transformation. Embrace them fully, and they will guide you toward a life of freedom, peace, and fulfillment.

What to Do If You've Decided to Walk Away from a Toxic Family Member
Deciding to walk away from a family member is incredibly difficult and often fraught with emotional turmoil. However, it can also be a necessary step toward preserving your mental health and reclaiming your life. If you have decided to cut ties with a toxic family member, remember that this decision is a testament to your courage and commitment to your well-being.

Walking away from a toxic relationship is not an admission of defeat but an act of profound self-care and self-respect. It signifies that you are choosing to prioritize your peace, happiness, and future over the chaos and pain of a harmful relationship. This journey may feel lonely at times, but remember that you are not alone. Many have walked this path and emerged stronger, and so can you.

In the face of such a challenging decision, self-care becomes more important than ever. Engage in activities that nurture your mind, body, and spirit. Whether it's through exercise, meditation, hobbies, or spending time in nature, find what rejuvenates you and makes it a regular part of your routine. Self-care is not selfish; it is essential for your healing and growth.

Seeking help when needed is also crucial. Professional support from therapists, counselors, or support groups can provide you with the tools and understanding needed to navigate this difficult period. They can offer guidance, validation, and strategies to help you cope with the emotions and challenges that arise from cutting ties with a family member.

Living in the present moment is a powerful practice. It involves acknowledging your thoughts and feelings without letting them dominate your experience. When thoughts about the past or fears about the future arise, gently bring your attention back to the now. This practice can help you find clarity and calm amidst the storm of emotions that walking away from a family member may stir up.

It is also essential to cultivate a support system of friends, mentors, and loved ones who understand and respect your decision. These individuals can provide emotional support, practical advice, and a sense of belonging during this transition. Surround yourself with people who uplift and encourage you, reminding you that you are valued and loved.

As you embark on this new chapter, embrace the freedom that comes with releasing toxic relationships. Celebrate your strength in making such a significant decision for your well-being. Use this time to rediscover yourself, your passions, and your dreams. Walking away from a toxic family member can open the door to new opportunities for growth and happiness.

Mindfulness can be a powerful ally during this time. By practicing mindfulness, you can stay grounded in the present moment, reducing anxiety and emotional overwhelm. Remember the words of Eckhart Tolle: "The past has no power over the present moment." When you focus on the present, you diminish the hold that past hurts and future worries have on you. Mindfulness encourages you to observe your thoughts without judgment, allowing you to let go of the people, thoughts, and circumstances that pull you away from the peace of the present moment.

Next Steps

As you move forward, embrace the profound journey of continued growth and transformation. The path you have walked thus far is a testament to your resilience, courage, and unwavering commitment to healing. The lessons and strategies you have learned are not just temporary measures; they are the foundational pillars of your new life. Hold them close to your heart and continue to apply them with diligence and intention.

Maintain your daily practice of affirmations and reflections. These simple yet powerful tools are essential in nurturing a positive and focused mindset. Each affirmation is a seed planted in the fertile soil of your soul, capable of blossoming into strength, confidence, and self-love. Daily reflections allow you to connect deeply with your inner self, fostering self-awareness and insight. Through this practice, you remain grounded in your truth and aligned with your highest aspirations.

Self-care is a sacred act of self-love and self-respect. Regularly revisit your self-care routines, ensuring that you are nurturing your mind, body, and spirit. Self-care is not a luxury; it is a necessity for your well-being and continued growth. Engage in activities that replenish your energy, bring you joy, and foster inner peace. Whether it's meditation, exercise, creative pursuits, or simply taking time to rest, honor your needs and make self-care a priority.

Setting and reassessing your goals is a dynamic process that keeps you aligned with your evolving values and aspirations. As you grow and change, so will your goals and dreams. Take time to reflect on what truly matters to you and adjust your goals accordingly. This practice ensures that you are always moving in a direction that resonates with your authentic self. Celebrate your achievements and set new milestones that challenge and inspire you.

Remain open to seeking support when needed. There is immense strength in acknowledging when you need help and reaching out to others. Be proactive in cultivating and maintaining your support network. Surround yourself with individuals who uplift, encourage, and support your growth. These relationships are vital sources of strength and inspiration, reminding you that you are not alone on this journey.

Embrace new opportunities for growth and learning with an open heart and mind. Life is a continuous journey of discovery, and each experience offers a chance to learn and evolve. Be curious and willing to step out of your comfort zone. Challenges are not obstacles but opportunities for growth. Approach them with flexibility and resilience, knowing that each challenge you overcome strengthens your spirit and deepens your wisdom.

Spiritual growth is an integral part of your journey. Connect with your inner self and the larger universe through practices that resonate with you. Whether it's prayer, meditation, spending time in nature, or engaging in spiritual study, these practices can provide a sense of purpose and connection that transcends the physical world. They remind you of the deeper meaning and interconnectedness of all life.

As you continue on this path, remember that growth is a lifelong journey. There will be moments of triumph and moments of challenge, but each step forward brings you closer to your true self. Embrace the process with patience, compassion, and an unwavering belief in your ability to transform your life. Your journey is unique, and every experience contributes to the tapestry of your growth and healing.

Stay committed to your path with a sense of wonder and gratitude. Celebrate your progress, no matter how small, and honor the incredible strength that has brought you this far. You have the power to create a life that reflects your deepest values and highest aspirations. Embrace each day as a new opportunity to grow, learn, and become the person you are meant to be.

In moments of doubt or difficulty, return to the wisdom and practices you have cultivated. They are your guiding light, illuminating the path forward. Trust in your journey and the transformative power within you. You are capable of achieving extraordinary things, and your continued growth is a testament to the limitless potential of the human spirit.

As you move forward, may you find peace, joy, and fulfillment in every step. Your journey is a sacred adventure, and each moment is an opportunity to deepen your connection with yourself and the world around you. Embrace your continued growth with an open heart, and know that the best is yet to come.

Final Thoughts
Each day presents a new opportunity to reinforce the positive

habits you have cultivated and to deepen your understanding of your true self. Embrace these opportunities with an open heart and a spirit filled with hope. Remember, every step forward, no matter how small, is a victory in itself. Your commitment to living authentically and embracing your true self is the foundation upon which your future will be built.

You possess an incredible strength and capability to thrive, no matter what challenges arise. This strength is your inner light, guiding you through the darkest moments and illuminating the path to a brighter, more fulfilling life. With each passing day, you are becoming more resilient, more compassionate, and more aligned with your true self. Hold on to this inner light and let it shine brightly, not only for yourself but also for those around you.

Imagine your future filled with supportive and loving relationships—people who see you for who you truly are and cherish your presence in their lives. These individuals are your inner circle, your tribe, and they are there to uplift and support you unconditionally. You are royalty in their eyes, deserving of respect, love, and admiration.

If your family doesn't treat you like a king or queen, then create a family of your own choosing, made up of people who care about your life, your future, and your interests as much as you do. Sometimes, all you need is one person to make that kind of family. Allow yourself to be surrounded by those who genuinely care for you and who celebrate your victories as their own. Always surround yourself with people who have your back and who genuinely care for you as much as they care for themselves.

As you move forward, keep your heart open to the endless possibilities that lie ahead. Your dreams are within reach, and your potential is boundless. Follow your heart with confidence, knowing that you have the power to create the life you envision. The road may not always be smooth, but with each step, you are carving out a path that is uniquely yours.

Stay true to yourself, for you are a remarkable individual with a unique purpose. Your authenticity is your greatest gift, and it is what will attract the right people and opportunities into your life. Embrace your journey with grace and determination, and let your spirit soar. You are capable of achieving greatness, and your story is one of resilience, strength, and triumph.

As you continue on this path, remember to nurture your inner circle and cultivate relationships that bring out the best in you. Surround yourself with those who uplift and inspire you, and let go of anything that no longer serves your highest good. Your well-being and happiness are paramount, and you deserve to be cherished and celebrated every day.

Thank you for allowing this book to be a part of your journey. It has been an honor to walk alongside you, sharing insights, reflections, and encouragement. May your continued growth be filled with joy, peace, and fulfillment. Here's to the bright future that lies ahead—a future where you are free to live authentically, follow your dreams, and shine your light for all to see.

Believe in yourself, embrace your journey, and celebrate the magnificent person you are becoming. The best is yet to come, and your future is as bright as your spirit. Here's to your ongoing transformation and the limitless possibilities that await you.

You are worthy, you are loved, and you are destined for greatness!

Steven Todd Bryant
Summer, 2024